SNAKE
OIL
SCIENCE

SNAKE
OIL
SCIENCE

*The Truth About
Complementary and
Alternative Medicine*

R. BARKER BAUSELL

OXFORD
UNIVERSITY PRESS

2007

OXFORD

UNIVERSITY PRESS

Oxford University Press, Inc., publishes works that further
Oxford University's objective of excellence
in research, scholarship, and education.

Oxford   New York
Auckland   Cape Town   Dar es Salaam   Hong Kong   Karachi
Kuala Lumpur   Madrid   Melbourne   Mexico City   Nairobi
New Delhi   Shanghai   Taipei   Toronto

With offices in
Argentina   Austria   Brazil   Chile   Czech Republic   France   Greece
Guatemala   Hungary   Italy   Japan   Poland   Portugal   Singapore
South Korea   Switzerland   Thailand   Turkey   Ukraine   Vietnam

Copyright © 2007 R. Barker Bausell

Published by Oxford University Press, Inc.
198 Madison Avenue, New York, New York 10016

www.oup.com

Oxford is a registered trademark of Oxford University Press

Library of Congress Cataloging-in-Publication Data
Bausell, R. Barker, 1942–
Snake oil science : the truth about complementary and alternative
medicine / by R. Barker Bausell.
p. cm.
Includes bibliographical references.
ISBN 978-0-19-531368-0
1. Alternative medicine.   2. Placebo (Medicine)   I. Title.
R733.B29 2007   615.5—dc22

1 3 5 7 9 8 6 4 2

Printed in the United States of America
on acid-free paper

To Rebecca Barker Bausell

CONTENTS

ACKNOWLEDGMENTS

I would like to acknowledge the efforts of Allison Hewitt for her help in acquiring many of the references used in this work, Sue Warga for copyediting the text, and Lelia Mander for supervising the book's production. Most of all I owe a debt of gratitude to Marion Osmun, my editor, who believed in the project and turned it into a far better book than it would have been otherwise. I am convinced that this project never would have come to fruition without her help, guidance, and encouragement.

In his delightful book *Voodoo Science: The Road from Foolishness to Fraud,* Dr. Robert Park provides an amusing firsthand account of a press conference called by the National Institutes of Health's then nascent Office of Alternative Medicine to lay out its scientific agenda. After describing some introductory remarks by a senator who had been instrumental in pressuring the NIH to establish the office in the first place (after reputedly having been cured of his allergies by bee pollen purchased from an individual who had claimed, among other things, that "the risen Jesus Christ, when he came back to Earth, consumed bee pollen"), Park went on to describe a type of behavior that I observed numerous times during my own involvement in an NIH-funded center for complementary and alternative research:

> Perhaps the strangest part of the press conference consisted of brief statements by individual members of the editorial review board of what they saw as the most important issues for the Office of Alternative Medicine [OAM]. One insisted that the number-one health problem in the Unites States is magnesium deficiency; another was convinced that the expanded use of acupuncture could revolutionize medicine; and so it went around the table, with each touting his or her preferred therapy. But there was no sense of conflict or rivalry. As each spoke, the other would nod in agreement. The purpose of the OAM, I began to realize, was to demonstrate that these disparate therapies all

work. It was my first glimpse of what it is that holds alternative medicine together: there is no internal dissent in a community that feels itself besieged from the outside.[1]

In my opinion Park's observations regarding the bonds that hold this community together are quite perceptive. I would add that another of the group's shared beliefs is that the validity of their therapies transcends conventional scientific methods altogether. As things turned out, however, the OAM (one of whose early directors was an unabashed advocate of homeopathy) mutated into the more prestigious National Center for Complementary and Alternative Medicine, which began funding high-quality, scientifically rigorous controlled clinical trials of complementary and alternative medical (CAM) therapies, which in turn helped introduce the evaluation of the effectiveness of CAM therapies into mainstream scientific thought. All of which, not unlike a metaphoric particle accelerator, provided the conditions for a crisis that has occurred many times in the history of science: a collision between science and belief.

Belief itself is a very personal human attribute that is extremely important to all of us. We believe in things for many reasons: because we want to, because we need to, because certain beliefs fit our worldviews or religious tenets, because the majority of our acquaintances share them, because of the advocacy of someone we respect, and perhaps most frequently of all because of how we interpret our personal experiences.

All of these can constitute perfectly reasonable bases upon which to found one's beliefs. All of these are also perfectly capable of leading to incorrect decisions about what is beneficial, what is ineffective, and what is downright harmful—especially when we are misled by those we trust.

This book describes another basis upon which to found certain types of beliefs, specifically those involved in ascertaining the *cause* of things. That basis depends on performing carefully controlled experiments designed to ascertain what helps us, what does not, and why. It is a wondrous process with one serious weakness: it is performed by people who are themselves sometimes unavoidably influenced by their beliefs, who sometimes aren't sufficiently trained, and—alas—who sometimes deceive the rest of us for their personal gain.

Still, of all the reasons people believe things, science is the most objective and the most immune from those logical and emotional frailties that define our humanity—especially when we take the quality of this scientific evidence into consideration. What this book is about, then, is the evaluation of the scientific research that has been conducted to assess the effectiveness of a large, catchall category of medical therapies variously referred to as complementary and alternative, unconventional, or integrative, such as acupuncture, herbs, and homeopathic remedies. Millions of people are increasingly using these therapies to supplement or replace an equally large category of therapies such as pharmaceuticals and surgery that are now considered to be the province of conventional medicine.

ABOUT YOUR AUTHOR

By training I am what is known as a research methodologist. Having long since resigned myself to watching people's eyes glaze over when I try to explain what this unwieldy job title entails, I now simply call myself a biostatistician. If anyone were to inquire further (which so far no one has), I would add that I specialize in the design of research studies that allow us to try out different approaches to problems, assign numbers to what happens, and then interpret these numbers in an objective manner. If I took myself a bit more seriously, I would add that I am also something akin to an empirical philosopher, studying the strategies that facilitate our species' ability to make correct inferences (or judgments).

But since there are no job descriptions (or jobs) for empirical philosophers, my ticket to direct deposit emanates from my specialization in those parts of the scientific process that allow us to decide what benefits people and what does not. Fortunately for me, over time carefully controlled research (such as randomized, controlled trials) involving numerical data has proved more dependable for showing us what works and what does not than has reliance upon expert opinions, experience, hunches, or the teachings of those we revere.

Unfortunately, this scientific, number-driven approach to knowledge also has some severe limitations. It cannot tell us what is ethically preferable or even what is best for us. It can only tell us if one discrete approach to accomplishing a specified task is superior, inferior, or equivalent to some other discrete approach. It is, in other words, a most excellent way to answer very specific, and very small, questions—questions, for example, that compare the effectiveness of two approaches for accomplishing one specific task, such as "Does drug A reduce AIDS patients' viral loads more than drug B?" The scientific approach cannot, however, go even a single step further to answer questions such as "What is the best way to reduce viral loads among HIV patients?" or "Is stem cell research justifiable?" And it is a completely ineffectual way to answer larger questions, such as "What is the meaning of life?" or "Does God exist?"

So what I suppose I really am is not a philosopher at all but merely a scientist, an experimenter, a designer of experiments, an analyzer of data, and an interpreter of these analyses. It was for these mundane purposes, at any rate, that I was recruited several years ago to apply my skills to the emerging field of evaluating CAM therapies.

While serving as the director of research at the University of Maryland's NIH-funded Complementary Medicine Program (now called the Center for Integrative Medicine), I had the opportunity to design and supervise the conduct of randomized clinical trials to ascertain if acupuncture and "mind-body" medicine could reduce pain and increase physical functioning for several medical conditions. I also read and evaluated hundreds of other CAM research reports. As informative as these experiences were, however, I believe the most enlightening aspects of my five-year exposure to the world of CAM research revolved around my increased intellectual interest in a phenomenon known as the placebo effect. It is this phenomenon (which is at least as interesting and counterintuitive as any New Age health practice) that holds the key to answering this book's pivotal question: whether or not CAM therapies work.

And while the placebo effect does not provide the complete answer to issues such as why so many people can be so sure that therapies such as homeopathy or acupuncture work for them (or why science is so impotent in supporting or refuting these beliefs), it does provide a starting point for their consideration. This is because the placebo effect is a prominent member of an extended family of logical, psychological, and physiological phenomena that conspire (separately and together) to confound our everyday thought processes—not to mention the results of even our most carefully conceived scientific experiments. And it is basically the circumvention of these impediments to clear thinking that has constituted my job description for the past thirty years.

ABOUT THIS BOOK

Because of its emphasis upon high-quality scientific evidence, this book could not have been written in April 1999, when I assumed my position at the aforementioned Complementary Medicine Program. Now, however, enough evidence has accumulated to permit the first scientific evaluation of complementary and alternative medicine. And that is what this book is about.

This book is also about explaining how such scientific evidence is generated in the first place, because without an understanding of the logic of experimentation, it is impossible to make sense of the huge morass of conflicting evidence with which the media is constantly barraging us about any number of therapies, CAM or conventional. Fortunately, this logic is simple, involving nothing more than comparing one group of individuals who receive a therapy with another group who *think* they are receiving that therapy.

But just because the logic of scientific experimentation is simple does not mean that it is simple to run a high-quality clinical trial. In fact, in a new area of endeavor such as CAM research, poorly conducted research constitutes the norm rather than the exception, and poorly conducted research almost inevitably produces false positive results—regardless of what is being evaluated. There are many reasons for this, but basically they are of two genres. The first involves impediments to logical thought that appear to be hardwired into our brains and that affect us all, scientists and nonscientists. These impediments are easily overcome through the proper application of scientific methods. The second is a bit more nefarious, involving several forms of bias that are capable of confounding the results obtained from even the most carefully controlled experiments. Such biases include unconsciously allowing our preconceived conceptions to influence our observations, failing to tell the whole truth, putting a positive spin on evidence in support of a cherished belief, succumbing to old-fashioned dishonesty, and, most common of all, simple incompetence.

So it really is not possible to evaluate evidence in an area such as complementary and alternative medicine without considering very seriously the quality of this evidence and how susceptible it is to bias. My goal in writing this book is to draw on my experience in designing, evaluating, and statistically analyzing all kinds of research—including that conducted in the closely knit, often overzealous world of CAM—to guide the uninitiated reader through the labyrinth of factors that often bias scientific research of this sort.

I believe it is a worthwhile journey, however, because its ultimate goal will be to answer the question not of whether complementary and alternative therapies work (because, as we'll discover, most *do* work—although weakly, temporarily, and for subjective outcomes) but of whether or not they work for the reasons their proponents claim. So in a sense this journey involves a search for understanding the cause of things, which is basically what science is all about.

Complementary and alternative medical therapies provide an unusually challenging vehicle for this journey, since most people believe that they already know the answer to this question. And soon, if current trends continue, the majority of Americans who can afford such treatments will be engaging in them. But what if all these people are wrong? One of my primary motivations for writing this book was to illustrate how such a scenario could occur. Another was to give people who depend upon the results of clinical trials to make major health decisions a basis for separating good research from pseudoscientific hype.

So what this book is about is the *science* of complementary and alternative medicine—not its politics or its philosophical basis, and not whether Oprah Winfrey advocates it. This book is about how this science is conducted, evaluated, and synthesized to arrive at a bottom-line conclusion about whether CAM therapies are effective. In the consideration of these issues, I pledge to be as frank, transparent, and dispassionately honest as is humanly possible. Fortunately, just because science values objectivity doesn't mean that science itself is in any way boring. Examining scientific evidence in order to determine whether something is effective or not is in many ways similar to solving a mystery or to taking an exciting journey into uncharted territory. And while I cannot guarantee that I will be able to convey this excitement, I do guarantee that the concepts I present will be thought-provoking and that my assessment of the evidence will be as objective as I can make it.

What I seek to do in this book, then, is to demonstrate how millions of intelligent people could be correct when they conclude that their symptoms were relieved as soon as they received a complementary and alternative medical treatment, but incorrect when they conclude that this relief was due to the treatment itself. I will argue, in fact, that the best scientific evidence available suggests that the genesis of this relief is something else entirely. And while this possibility may seem counterintuitive, I will suggest that this "something else" is actually the placebo effect, a phenomenon recognized at least since the time of Hippocrates and used by physicians ever since.

The evidence that will be considered in this book primarily revolves around whether there is such a thing as a placebo effect and whether or not there are complementary and alternative medical effects that operate independently of it. Indeed, the primary question to which this book is dedicated to answering is:

Is any complementary and alternative medical therapy more effective than a placebo?

To answer this question, I will have to explain exactly what constitutes a complementary and alternative medical therapy as well as a placebo. I will then have to convince you, the reader, that not only are your personal experiences with CAM largely irrelevant for answering questions such as this, but so are those of your physicians and your CAM therapists. I don't think you will have much difficulty accepting this proposition once you meet the other members of the placebo effect's extended family that I mentioned previously, whose sole reason for existence sometimes appears to be to make fools of us all—especially when it comes to figuring out *why* things happen the way they do. I also don't believe that you will need much convincing that not all scientific research can be accepted at face value either. Or that research results based upon high-quality studies are more credible than those based upon poor-quality work. Or that research results that are consonant with findings from other scientific disciplines tend to be more plausible than those that have no basis other than their authors' personal beliefs. Or that research that does not control for the placebo effect and its relatives, whether designed to evaluate complementary and alternative therapies or the latest conventional drugs, almost always produces false positive results (namely, that whatever is being evaluated is effective).

Once these preliminary issues have been addressed, then we can examine the actual scientific studies that address four specific issues:

1. Is there such a thing as a placebo effect? In other words, can a completely bogus therapy work?
2. Is there something that has been demonstrated to take place within the body that could explain how a placebo effect occurs? In other words, if there is evidence that a placebo effect exists,

are these results consonant with findings from other scientific disciplines?

3. Is there such a thing as a CAM effect over and above what can be attributed to the placebo effect?

4. Is there something that has been demonstrated to take place within the body that could explain how one or more of these CAM effects occurs? Again, this addresses the issue of whether or not the existing evidence is consistent with what we know about the biology of the human body.

Then, based upon the answers to these four questions, I will provide as definitive an answer as is scientifically possible at this point in time to our original question—which is important enough to repeat: *Is any complementary and alternative medical therapy more effective than a placebo?*

SNAKE
OIL
SCIENCE

CHAPTER ONE

The Rise of Complementary and Alternative Therapies

In the early 1990s, people whose job it was to study trends in health care began to notice the emergence of a strange phenomenon: ordinary people appeared to be turning en masse to what were variously termed "alternative," "unconventional," "New Age," "complementary," "complementary and alternative," or "integrative" medical practitioners. True, some conventional physicians and their organizations likened these practices to eighteenth- and nineteenth-century medical charlatanism stereotypically practiced from the backs of medicine wagons. But in truth many of these complementary and alternative medicine advocates practiced under the auspices (and blessings) of our most prestigious medical schools, such as those at Harvard and Stanford. They presented themselves with impeccable professional decorum, invoking science as the basis of their practices, reassuring their audiences that their research was funded by the National Institutes of Health, and publishing their articles in prestigious mainstream medical journals.

Of course, some of their colleagues still came across as snake oil sellers, but if institutions such as Harvard Medical School and the National Institutes of Health endorsed such practices, who was to say that medical charlatanism was at work here? After all, such practices hadn't been a significant public health issue since medicine's golden age had ushered in antibiotics, ever more effective vaccines, chemotherapies, refined surgical procedures, extremely sensitive high-tech diagnostic procedures, and a multibillion-dollar multinational pharmaceutical industry that appeared to have a pill for every conceivable health complaint—every health complaint, that is, except the most common ones: symptoms due to chronic, non–life-threatening illnesses that drastically affected their victims' quality of life.

For these, medical science's answers left a great deal to be desired. No vaccine existed to prevent arthritis, surgery was largely ineffective for chronic back problems, and nowhere in the bewildering variety of pharmaceutical products was there a pain medication that could be taken 365 days a year without eventually causing side effects as problematic as the symptoms it was designed to eliminate. Also, with pharmaceutical marketing came the expectation that a medical answer did exist for just about every human complaint. Indeed, sometimes even the complaints themselves were invented in order to sell the solution, such as Miles Laboratories' successful marketing of the "blahs" as something that Alka-Seltzer could cure.

So, in a sense, medical science's truly impressive twentieth-century successes may be indirectly responsible for this migration toward alternative health care providers. After all, it was undeniable that more people were living longer due to these medical achievements; ergo, more people were afflicted by the conditions that accompanied the aging process. Also, as people (especially in the more affluent segments of society) had more leisure time to concentrate on their health conditions, they became increasingly sensitized to symptoms (physical, mental, and psychosomatic) that they felt they should not have to deal with on an everyday basis.

Along with these symptoms came "new" diseases—such as chronic fatigue syndrome and fibromyalgia—for which biochemical or radiological diagnostic tests had not yet been developed, which in turn meant that a biochemical solution was not on the horizon. Then, to make matters worse, some physicians began to question the very existence of any conditions that could not be associated with a specific biomarker.

Confounding all of this was a growing consumer movement that increasingly expected high-quality, respectful service—an expectation that fit poorly with both medical paternalism (which sometimes appeared to view patients more as potentially misbehaving children than as consumers) and the emerging managed care model (which did view patients as consumers, but ones whose health needs were generic and hence could be treated quickly, efficiently, and relatively impersonally).

We have, in short, entered an era of consumer dissatisfaction with conventional medicine's inability to treat, much less fix, chronic, sometimes disabling aches and pains. But, for better or worse, dissatisfaction tends to create demand, which in turn is met by supply. And in this case, what was being supplied was a truly bewildering variety of therapies, the vast majority of whose practitioners approached medical care from a holistic, nonbiological, nonpharmacological, noninvasive, non-evidence-based, nonscientific perspective. Some borrowed their approaches from ancient forms of medical treatment derived from the Far East, such as acupuncture (China), ayurvedic medicine (India), or kampo (Japan). Others were based upon more recently developed approaches such as homeopathic or chiropractic medicine, while still others adopted a naturalistic worldview that assumed the cure for (or prevention of) all disease resided in natural processes already in the body or available from nature. The one thing all of these therapeutic approaches had in common, however, was that none had a conventional scientific basis, nor were any (despite the protestations of university-based "alternative scientists") based upon what a conventional scientist would label as "hard" evidence.

There is no requirement that something like a CAM therapy should be constrained by scientific evidence or even by the scientific paradigm, for that matter. Many mainstream medical procedures are performed without sufficient scientific evidence. Miles Laboratories certainly wasn't required to prove that the "blahs" really existed, much less that Alka-Seltzer was an effective treatment for them. Countless surgical procedures have come and gone over the past few decades without ever having been subjected to controlled scientific scrutiny. In addition, all of us engage in certain superstitious behaviors simply because we enjoy them or because they provide us with some degree of hope or feeling of control over our destiny. So who is to draw the line between legitimacy and charlatanism? Pharmaceutical companies? Physicians? CAM therapists?

The answer is: anyone who understands what constitutes scientific evidence and what the difference is between science and pseudoscience. In the final analysis, the scientific evaluation of a therapy's effectiveness is ultimately not a matter of opinion, nor is it a function of who shouts the loudest or who garners the most votes or who is the best salesperson. And ultimately, most ordinary people really do want to know whether there is scientific evidence supporting the effectiveness of the medical therapies they receive (and pay for). So in this spirit, let's first examine the scientific evidence surrounding the use of CAM therapies to see if CAM truly is a phenomenon of sufficient magnitude to even merit serious scientific scrutiny.

THE EXTENT OF PUBLIC USE OF CAM THERAPIES

Surveys conducted to ascertain how many people use CAM therapies (and for what purposes they use them) have been performed by two types of investigators: CAM and governmental. As would be expected, the former generally provide larger estimates than the latter, with the most frequently cited of the CAM surveys arriving at the counterintuitive claim that CAM therapy visits now surpass the "total visits to all US primary care physicians."[1] But even the higher-quality surveys (in terms of numbers of respondents, how these respondents were selected, and the objectivity of the questions) conducted by the federal government's National Center for Health Statistics and the prestigious Robert Wood Johnson Foundation still point to a very high incidence of CAM use in the United States.[2]

The first of the federal surveys, the 1996 National Health Survey, interviewed a total of 16,038 adults (which was several times the number contained in all of the previous surveys conducted by CAM researchers combined).[3] The second survey, conducted three years later, involved almost twice as many people (30,801) and produced some truly staggering estimates (Table 1.1), such as the fact that almost 15 million Americans had visited a chiropractor during the past year and 19 million had employed herbal remedies.[4]

And then three years after that, in 2002, another governmental survey of more than 30,000 people (Table 1.2) found that 36 percent of the American public had used some form of non-prayer-based CAM therapy during the past twelve months.[5]

Table 1.1. Proportion of the Adult Population of the United States Using CAM Therapies During the Past Twelve Months, 1999

CAM Therapy	Percentage of the U.S. Population Using the Therapy	Number of U.S. Adults Using the Therapy
Spiritual healing or prayer	13.7%	26,997,000
Herbal medicine	9.6%	18,937,000
Chiropractic therapy	7.6%	14,969,000
Massage therapy	6.4%	12,539,000
Relaxation therapy	5.0%	9,891,000
Homeopathy	3.1%	6,182,000
Imagery	1.7%	3,370,000
Acupuncture	1.4%	2,691,000
Energy healing (e.g., Reiki)	1.1%	2,142,000
Hypnosis	0.5%	1,013,000
Biofeedback	0.5%	1,029,000

Table 1.2. Proportion of the Adult Population of the United States Using CAM Therapies During the Past Twelve Months, 2002

CAM Therapy	Percentage of the U.S. Population Using the Therapy	Number of U.S. Adults Using the Therapy
Natural products (e.g., herbs)*	18.9%	38,183,000
Deep breathing exercises	11.6%	23,457,000
Meditation	7.6%	15,336,000
Chiropractic therapy	7.5%	15,226,000
Yoga	5.1%	10,386,000
Massage therapy	5.0%	10,052,000
Progressive relaxation	3.0%	6,185,000
Megavitamin therapy	2.8%	5,749,000
Guided imagery	2.1%	4,194,000
Homeopathy	1.7%	3,433,000
Tai chi	1.3%	2,565,000
Acupuncture	1.1%	2,136,000
Energy healing (e.g., Reiki)	0.5%	1,080,000
Qi gong	0.3%	527,000
Hypnosis	0.2%	505,000
Naturopathy	0.2%	498,000
Biofeedback	0.1%	278,000
Folk medicine	0.1%	233,000
Ayurvedic medicine	0.1%	154,000
Chelation therapy	0.01%	66,000

* Does not include vitamins and minerals

TYPES OF CAM THERAPIES

While there is no question that there are a lot of people out there using CAM therapies, what specifically are these practices and why does the government (as well as their practitioners) refer to them as "complementary and alternative" therapies? The answer is not as simple as it appears because the individual therapies (such as acupuncture) and the categories of therapies (such as energy healing) listed in these governmental surveys represent only the tip of an iceberg consisting of hundreds of options marketed by legions of therapists. So before attempting to define exactly what is meant by the term "complementary and alternative medicine," let me first offer a very broad look at the field itself by attempting to categorize this mélange as meaningfully as possible.

Perhaps the clearest way to approach this daunting task is to conceptualize the modalities listed in Tables 1.1 and 1.2 as belonging to (or emanating from) the following five categories: (1) indigenous medical systems, (2) recently developed (nonindigenous) medical systems, (3) spiritual or energetic healing techniques, (4) methods of relaxation, and (5) extensions of conventional scientific findings. And while some therapies arguably belong to more than one of these categories, their use provides us with a broad, succinct gestalt of the entire field.

Indigenous Medical Systems

By indigenous medical systems, I mean the collection of healing practices that gradually developed in ancient cultures prior to the explosion of biochemically grounded medical techniques in Europe and America during the nineteenth and twentieth centuries. As would be expected, these older systems relied heavily upon locally available flora, external manipulation of the body (since surgery, except for the most traumatic of injuries, was usually out of the question), elaborate ceremonies (which appeared to be designed, whether consciously or not, to impart curative expectations), and basically anything else available from the environment that could be considered to have healing properties.

The philosophical bases of a number of these systems, not to mention their noninvasive approach to healing, have become relatively attractive to many people in recent years. As a result of this popularity, a number have "medical colleges" and schools devoted to training new practitioners (both in their countries of origin and in the West).

When most of us hear the term "complementary and alternative medicine," we usually think of individual therapies (such as acupuncture, massage, yoga, or herbal therapy) that were originally developed within these indigenous systems rather than the systems themselves. Many of these therapies have changed drastically since their original conception and have mutated into a number of different philosophic approaches. Still, a brief look at a few of these medical paradigms is a useful starting point—especially since modern science has a tendency to narrow things down to their simplest unit, while the proponents of CAM therapies prefer to take a much broader, holistic approach.

Thus while the uninitiated tend to look at a procedure such as acupuncture as a discrete set of behaviors involving placing thin needles into selected body parts, in reality there are actually many different types of acupuncture (such as Chinese, Japanese, medical, and auricular, to name just a few) that employ diverse techniques, have different proposed mechanisms of action, and are accompanied by varied (complementary) therapies. Let's begin with one of the oldest, if not *the* oldest, medical system of which we are aware: traditional Chinese medicine.

Traditional Chinese Medicine

The overall theory, purpose, or paradigm governing traditional Chinese medicine (TCM) is that the most effective way to address a patient's symptoms is by restoring the balance of two properties within the body, called *yin* and *yang,* which are both opposite and complementary to one another.[6]

Yin generally represents properties variously described (recognizing limitations inherent in translation across both language and culture) as "female," "inactive," "internal," "cold," and "dark," while yang represents "male," "active," "external," "hot," and "bright" properties. Lack of balance between the two is considered to be a primary cause of illness; hence the underlying purpose of TCM medical treatment is to bring yin and yang back into balance via the manipulation of their physical manifestations: *qi* (or *chi*), the body's vital energy (yang), which generates and drives its mother, blood (yin).

Based upon a complex diagnostic system in which traditional practitioners are able to determine exactly what is out of balance and what is not by feeling patients' (noncardiovascular) pulses or examining their tongues, a combination of several potential therapies may be prescribed, each category of which has a different function. Some of the more important of these strategies include:

- **Herbs**, which are also employed by every other indigenous medical system known. Chinese herbal formulas tend to be combinations of at least four individual herbs (usually administered as a tea or broth) and can be traced back to at least the third century B.C., when 280 formulas were recorded in the Ma Wang Tui tomb document, a number that reputedly increased to more than 60,000 by A.D. 1644.[7]

- **Massage**, also a popular ancient medical strategy, which is used to balance yin and yang as well as to loosen joints, relax muscles, restore a fuller range of motion to limbs, and reduce pain.

- **Qi gong**, which is a form of meditation combined with gentle body movements designed to achieve a normal balance of body movement. A later variant, *tai chi,* was originally developed as a martial art and is believed to balance yin and yang. (Yet another variant is external qi gong, in which a qi gong master is believed to be able to direct the flow of qi through other people's bodies by using his or her own energies.)

- **Acupuncture**, which may have been developed in China as much as four millennia ago and is practiced by placing extremely thin needles at selected points along channels connecting different parts of the body called meridians, through which qi flows. The needles, among other things, regulate this flow of energy and help ensure a balance between yin and yang, thereby curing a number of diseases or ameliorating their symptoms.

Of these four TCM treatment components, acupuncture is the most widely used outside of China. (Herbal therapies are much more commonly employed in general, but not necessarily classical Chinese formulations.) There are, in fact, a number of acupuncture variations even in TCM, including moxibustion (in which a specific herb is burned above the skin or actually on an acupuncture point in order to facilitate the unimpeded flow of qi through the appropriate meridians). Pressure (called acupressure) is also sometimes substituted for actual needle insertion.

Outside China, acupuncture, like many other ancient therapies, has been adapted and changed. The Japanese have developed their own technique involving shallower needle insertion, while European, American, and modern Chinese practitioners have added such innovations as connecting an electrical source to their stainless-steel needles (called electro-acupuncture) in order to maximize their effects.

Acupuncture-like machines have also been invented, which deliver electrical current directly to selected points (sometimes at classical acupuncture points, sometimes at other locations called trigger points) with or without the use of needles. These particular therapies (called, depending upon the method of administering the electrical impulses, transcutaneous electrical nerve stimulation [TENS] or pericutaneous electrical nerve stimulation [PENS]) have a more physiologically based rationale (which I'll discuss in Chapter 13) that has now also been adopted by many modern acupuncture researchers as well as a number of other CAM therapies.

Ayurvedic Medicine

Ayurvedic medicine is another ancient medical system that has witnessed some increase in popularity during the latter part of the twentieth century. Originating in India, it is reputed to be older even than TCM. From the words *ayur* (meaning "life") and *veda* ("knowledge" or "science"), this system is as much concerned with philosophical and spiritual issues as medical ones and, as such, is deeply influenced by the unique Indian view of the origin of life and its meaning.[8]

Ayurvedic medicine bears some superficial similarities to traditional Chinese medicine. As one example, it posits three complementary and opposing forms of energy (*vata, pitta,* and *kasha*) that cause disease when not in balance, just as is true of yin and yang. Ayurvedic treatments, however, have relatively little in common with those of their Chinese cousin and include such practices as therapeutic vomiting, purgatives/laxatives, medicated enemas, bloodletting, herbs (although fewer in number than in TCM), yoga, and chromotherapy (the use of colored lights or wearing clothing of prescribed colors keyed to the ailment).

Native American Medicine

While quite diverse, given the hundreds of independent nations (or tribes) that shared North America before the European invasion, Native American medical systems often involve prayers, chants, songs, drumbeats, cleansing via smudging the patient with the smoke of (among other things) sacred plants, the use of herbs, therapeutic touch (laying on of hands), and the performance of various ceremonial rites.[9] Not widely adopted outside the Native American community, the paradigmatic importance that many of these medical and philosophical systems place upon environmental balance and natural forces has nevertheless recently made them more attractive, if not commonly practiced.

Tibetan Medicine

Tibetan medicine is another politically and spiritually appealing indigenous medical system for some people, although its individual therapies are also not commonly practiced. Influenced by its ayurvedic predecessor (as well as Buddhist and pre-Buddhist philosophy), its unique mechanism of action posits three universal elements: *chi* (space), *schara* (energy), and *badahan* (matter). These three elements are not conceived as existing independently of one another, although any individual is more likely to be influenced by one than by another and these relative balances have important clinical and therapeutic implications.[10] Treatments themselves include (but are not limited to) herbal formulas, nutritional prescriptions (in which taste plays an important role, as do seasonal adjustments), and a unique form of massage that can include abdominal, spinal, head, and neck manipulation.

The physician-patient relationship plays an especially important role in Tibetan therapy, as does the concept of what is (poorly) translated as the "subtle body," which is a network of channeling structures designed to carry a form of psychic energy that is crucial to the body's health. This network runs parallel to, but is distinct from, the actual physiological networks that carry nutrition (blood vessels) and electrical impulses (the nervous system). Various preventive and therapeutic strategies exist to facilitate the flow of psychic energy through the subtle body, one example of which is the insertion of a needle covered with a vegetable-based, combustible substance that is lit to remove energy blockages and redirect the flow of this energy.

Nonindigenous Medical Systems

Many of the individual therapies listed in Table 1.2 can be visualized as belonging to relatively new (but nonetheless full-fledged) medical systems that have grown up around their practice. The more popular ones have their own medical schools and have evolved philosophies and provider-patient "rules of engagement" that transcend the individual therapies upon which they are based. They, like their ancient predecessors, tend to be based not upon one individual therapy but rather upon a distinct philosophy of how the body responds to and prevents illness.

Osteopathic Medicine

Founded in the latter part of the nineteenth century by Andrew Taylor Still, a conventional physician, osteopathy was originally conceived as an expansion of conventional medical practice. As time went on (and perhaps as a result of conventional medicine's antipathy to this upstart and potential competitor), osteopathic medicine became more and more differentiated from its allopathic (conventional) counterpart. Osteopathic medical schools award a D.O. degree rather than an M.D. and, while embracing conventional anatomical and physiological concepts, it originally eschewed drugs and instead relied heavily upon physical manipulation.[11]

Unlike many CAM systems, though, this original philosophical approach changed as conventional medicine developed ever more effective therapies, so that osteopaths now have no problem prescribing, say, antibiotics in conjunction with whatever CAM therapy they prefer. Still, while osteopathy is difficult to classify because of its eclecticism, modern osteopathic physicians rely much more heavily upon physical techniques in both diagnosis and treatment than conventional medicine does. And if the following osteopathic physician's description of the treatment of an athletically induced sprained ankle is typical of the profession, then osteopaths are most definitely CAM providers:

> Before any other intervention is done the physician cradles the proximal aspects of the tibia and fibula in one hand and grasps both malleolae in the other. He or she holds them in a state of balanced, ligamentous tension, feeling the release of the strain-sprain take place. When the tissues feel palpably normalized the physician retests motion. The usual result is immediate: alleviation of dysfunctional symptoms.[12]

In osteopathic practice, manual treatments are believed to cure a much wider range of conditions than simple musculoskeletal complaints. Cranial manipulation (which was originally used primarily to correct cranial bone "restrictions" but has been extended to other parts of the body, such as the sacrum, where therapists use their hands to "listen" for restrictions or strains in the body), for example, is believed to benefit children with attention deficit disorder or developmental problems and is even performed on infants. Regardless of the therapy employed or the condition treated, however, osteopaths oppose treating symptoms only, considering the body to be a smoothly functioning unit that contains its own self-protecting and self-healing mechanisms, which can be gently accessed by a skillful practitioner.

Naturopathic Medicine

Also possessing their own medical schools and licensure structure, naturopathic proponents place most of their emphasis upon the body's ability to heal itself.[13] The discipline was officially initiated by Benedict Lust in 1902 but owes many of its tenets to the Chinese, Indian, and even Greek systems that date back thousands of years.

Naturopaths believe that healing (as well as the prevention of disease) occurs as a function of avoiding refined, non-organically-grown foods, avoiding stress, engaging in regular exercise, maintaining a positive outlook on life, and avoiding exposure to environmental toxins, among other things. Naturopathic physicians are not opposed, however, to using conventional radiological and laboratory diagnostic technologies as well as some less conventional ones (such as the assessment of nutritional status and digestive/eliminative functions).

While naturopaths stress a preventive lifestyle consonant with (although more elaborate than) recommendations of most present-day medical physicians, their prescribed treatments vary dramatically. Depending upon the practitioner's training and preferences, a naturopath may employ homeopathic remedies, herbal prescriptions, acupuncture, hydrotherapy, electromagnetic stimulation, detoxification, and just about any other CAM treatment yet invented.

Homeopathy

Originated by a German clinician named Samuel Hahnemann in the nineteenth century, this therapy was built upon two overriding principles. The first, that of "similars" or "like cures like," held that the best substance to cure a symptom was one that could induce that symptom in healthy subjects. The second held that homeopathic remedies actually become stronger as they are diluted, as long as this dilution is accompanied by succussion (a carefully prescribed vigorous shaking of the mixture in a special manner).[14] The final product is so diluted, in fact, that in many cases not a single molecule of the original substance would be expected to survive in the final product, which is important since many homeopathic remedies start out with toxic intent (e.g., the active ingredient in poison oak or the protective discharge emanating from the cuttlefish). The remaining substance is believed to possess the "memory" of what it started out as, but without its original toxicity.

Homeopaths also place much more emphasis upon developing a positive, caring relationship with their patients than do most conventional practitioners, and they probably spend more time with patients as well, trying to understand both the patient and the genesis of his or her illness. Homeopathy is also a complete medical system possessing its own schools, specialized journals, and a cadre of researchers and writers who have written enough books on the topic to fill a small library.

Chiropractic

The genesis of this medical system, the most popular of all CAM therapies, dates back to Daniel Palmer's alleged healing of a deaf individual by manually aligning his spinal column.[15] Palmer went on to establish the first chiropractic school in 1898, and since then chiropractic manipulation has become the most commonly practiced individual therapy in the United States.

Chiropractic manipulation itself is based upon the concept that many human illnesses arise from what is called subluxation (abnormal positioning or alignment) of the spine, and its hypothesized mechanism of action is largely based upon a conventional view of the nervous system and its importance in health. Philosophically, chiropractors (like so many other CAM therapists) believe that the body has an innate ability to heal itself and that one of the primary barriers to this ability, if not *the* primary barrier, resides in these subluxations within the various joints. Chiropractic practice therefore largely involves finding these abnormalities (and, like naturopathy, is not opposed to employing conventional, high-tech diagnostic procedures) and correcting them through manual manipulation.

Spiritual/Energy Healing

This category subsumes an extremely large number of individual therapies, all of which have two things in common: (1) a therapist with a special intent to heal and (2) a posited energy source that either emanates from this healer to the patient or resides somewhere else but can be channeled and controlled by the healer through a special gift (or in some cases through a technique that can be learned).

In an excellent overview of these therapies, the physician Daniel Benor argues that "spiritual healing is probably the oldest recognized therapy, used in some form in every known culture."[16] Many of the therapists who practice in this field are also believed to be expert diagnosticians who can detect the presence of disease through touch or the interpretation of auras emanating from their patients. Such therapists are also reported to sometimes have visible auras dramatically emanating from their bodies that other people.

Examples of some of these therapeutic genres include:

- **Shamanism**, which is stereotypically depicted in film as the heavily feathered Native American medicine man dancing around his patient, although there are many variations on this theme that do not cross into indigenous medical systems.

- **Therapeutic touch**, which was originally popularized by a nurse teaching at New York University and is now practiced by thousands of present-day nurses. It involves the concept of the healer centering his or her thoughts upon the sole purpose of healing the patient while holding his or her hands a few inches away from the patient's body.

- **Distant healing**, which can theoretically be accomplished by "intercessors" and often needs no more than the person's name to accomplish the healing. As implied by the therapy's name, it does not matter how far away the recipient is from the healer. In fact, it often doesn't even matter whether the patient knows the therapist, believes in the therapy, or is aware that he or she is being "treated."

- **Intuitive diagnostics**, which involves individuals who are believed to sense disharmonies and actual physical malfunctions in the body by touching or observing the patient, or by holding their hands near the patient's body. For especially gifted individuals, intuitive diagnostics can even occur from a distance. Other practices involve bodily maps in which, among other anatomical parts, the ear (auricular acupuncture), iris of the eye (iridology), and foot (reflexology) are believed to contain direct connections to every body part.

Spiritual or energetic therapists can be found in a number of cultures and within a number of different CAM systems. They include faith healers, who normally operate within a religious system and require the patient to share the same beliefs; Reiki masters, who can channel their energies to heal others and do not require any belief on the part of the patient; external qi gong practitioners, who do much the same thing; and a bewilderingly wide range of other practitioners, who often learn their healing techniques through coursework.

Relaxation-Oriented Therapies

The best-known examples of this genre of therapies are undoubtedly transcendental meditation (which belongs to a Vedic-inspired category of meditation that concentrates on a single thought or mantra) and mindfulness meditation (which has Buddhist origins and concentrates more on breathing and allowing the mind to simply observe rather than focus on whatever presents itself). Sometimes these procedures are advocated as a lifestyle or stress reduction technique (in which case they do not qualify as CAM), and sometimes they are prescribed for specific medical problems (in which case they do).

Other, more modern examples include progressive muscle relaxation, where the patient learns to tense and relax one muscle at a time, progressing throughout the body; deep breathing therapy, which is used not only as a relaxation method but also to reduce pain and promote healing and is a component of a number of other therapies such as yoga and meditation; meditation, which possesses many therapeutic forms and is hypothesized to have many healing properties in addition to bringing about simple relaxation and stress reduction; and guided imagery, which involves using one's imagination to reduce pain or promote healing.

Therapies Translated from (but Which Extend) Conventional Science

Examples in this category include chelation, biofeedback, and miscellaneous "natural drugs" whose constituents are known to be essential to bodily function and maintenance.

Chelation is based upon a conventional chemical action of a class of compounds known to incorporate ions of certain heavy metals (such as lead, which of course is extremely toxic) into their own atomic structure, thereby removing (or chelating) them from the body. When used for this purpose, chelation is not a CAM therapy, but when used to remove other harmful ions, such as those associated with fatty acids, it is.

Biofeedback as a therapy often employs the use of monitoring equipment to teach the individual to become attuned to his or her physiological functions (e.g., heart rate, electrical activity in the brain, skin temperature) and ultimately control them in the absence of any equipment.[17] It is based upon conventional scientific evidence that some physiological parameters, such as galvanic skin resistance, can be conditioned. When applied to the treatment of specific medical conditions (e.g., hypertension), however, this approach crosses the line into CAM.

"Natural drugs" is a descriptor that can encompass a host of substances such as glucosamine sulfate, which has been identified by science as one of the building blocks of cartilage and is therefore hypothesized to reduce joint pain and improve joint function when ingested. Substances sometimes called nutraceuticals, because they blur the line between nutrients and pharmaceuticals, might also be placed in this category. I do not discuss routine nutritional practices such as ingesting vitamins, minerals, fish oil, and other nutrients for health and medicinal purposes in this book because they are not normally conceptualized as CAM therapies.

DEFINITIONS OF CAM

It has been suggested that the diversity of these therapies argues against lumping them all under a single rubric such as "alternative," "complementary and alternative," or "integrative." I disagree, and so do most (though not all) of their practitioners. Indeed, most view their therapies as alternatives to conventional medical treatment, and most, as mentioned earlier, consider themselves as part of a common community that usually (but by no means always) stresses treatments that employ physiologic mechanisms of action currently unknown to biological science; are holistic in nature; are noninvasive, natural, and nontoxic; are applicable to an extremely wide range of medical conditions; and are individualized for each patient. Perhaps more important, in comparison with conventional medical providers, many (but again not all) of these practitioners tend to place less value on scientific evidence, often arguing that standard scientific methods are inadequate to evaluate the effectiveness of the treatments they offer.

Ultimately, however, whether or not it is reasonable to describe so many therapies using the same term is not crucially important, because the research we will review in this book is quite specific—dealing with the effects of specific therapies upon specific outcomes for specific diseases. And after reviewing this evidence, if it turns out that most of these disparate therapies do in fact produce the same results, and if these results can be explained by the same biological mechanism, then perhaps it will be reasonable to conclude that they do all belong together.

That said, any term used to describe such a diverse field will ultimately prove difficult to define. Even the CAM research community has struggled with the definition for some time, including the five years that I was associated with it. In fact, the original name of the field was "alternative medicine," which rubbed the conventional medical community the wrong way and generated more controversy than either academic proponents of these therapies or NIH administrators wanted. Other terms have been floated, including the now popular "integrative medicine" moniker, but the therapies and their philosophical bases have remained the same.

Regardless of labels, the *concept* itself has been defined in a politically correct way as "diagnosis, treatment and/or prevention which complements mainstream medicine by contributing to a common whole, satisfying a demand not met by orthodoxy, or diversifying the conceptual framework of medicine" or as "medical interventions not taught widely at U.S. medical schools or generally available at U.S. hospitals."[18] It could be defined even more vaguely as those therapies that patients are uncomfortable discussing with their doctors.

To make things just a bit more complicated, as hinted at in the preceding section, it is important to keep in mind what the *M* stands for in CAM. When used to increase flexibility or to reduce stress by facilitating relaxation, for example, yoga would not be considered a CAM therapy. Should yoga be employed to reduce pain due to a specific medical condition, however, then it would qualify as a CAM therapy because it is being used in this application as a *medical* treatment. The same is true of lifestyle diets, such as Atkins, vegetarian, or macrobiotic. When they are used to lose weight, to make people feel better about themselves, or for philosophic reasons, they are not CAM therapies; they may or may not be effective for these purposes, but either way they don't qualify as CAM. When they are used to treat a specific disorder such as arthritis, however, I would classify any type of diet as a CAM therapy unless it involved either deleting a specific substance proven by scientific research to be associated with a specific disease (such as salt for hypertension) or adding such a substance to prevent a specific medical disorder (such as folic acid for prenatal complications).

By the same token, I wouldn't classify people who pray for relief of a symptom or deliverance from a disease (or who ask other people to do so for them) as CAM users because prayer isn't a medical (i.e., physical, mental, chemical, or psychic) intervention. I would, however, classify someone who seeks out a provider who claims to be able to channel any sort of bodily, psychic, spiritual, or physical energy for medical purposes as a CAM user and the person so sought as a CAM provider.

Still, none of these definitions or disclaimers is completely satisfactory, so perhaps a more sensible approach is to keep in mind the gestalt of therapies listed in Tables 1.1 and 1.2 and simply proceed with the understanding that:

> *CAM therapies are physical, mental, chemical, or psychic interventions such as acupuncture, homeopathy, naturopathy, chelation, folk medicine, herbs, megavitamin therapy, nutraceuticals, chiropractic manipulation, massage, biofeedback, hypnosis, yoga, tai chi, qi gong, and any sort of energetic, psychic, or spiritual healing used for the treatment of specific medical conditions or disease symptoms. They are practiced in the absence of both scientific evidence proving their effectiveness and a plausible biological explanation for why they should be effective, and their practice continues unabated even after (1) there is scientific evidence that they are ineffective and (2) their biological basis is discredited.*

Now, this definition, while certainly more wordy, is not much more precise than any of its predecessors. What it also does is provide a means of making a crucial distinction between ineffective conventional medical practices and CAM therapies. There is a long list of medical and surgical procedures that have been abandoned during the past century when it became apparent that they weren't working as advertised, but few if any of these procedures were based upon entire physiological systems or physical forces that the average high school science teacher already knew didn't exist. And while there is no question that many other conventional medical procedures are still being practiced that haven't been subjected to rigorous scientific tests (and probably aren't effective), they will most likely be abandoned when shown to be completely ineffective or when it becomes apparent that another approach is more effective.

True, some surgeons may have performed their favorite procedures (or some internists may have prescribed a medication) longer than they should in the face of negative evidence, but in general most medical practitioners believe in the scientific process and value the evidence that it produces. In the face of definitive evidence, such as the recently conducted controlled trial that found knee surgery for osteoarthritis to be no more effective than a sham (placebo) surgical incision, most surgeons would be expected to eventually stop performing this particular operation.[19] I seriously doubt, however, that there is a traditional Chinese medicine practitioner anywhere who ever stopped performing acupuncture on an afflicted body part in the presence of similarly definitive negative evidence. CAM therapists simply do not value (and most, in my experience, do not understand) the scientific process.

Nevertheless, CAM therapies, like any other intervention, can be and have been subjected to scientific investigation, and a growing body of evidence has accumulated to answer the question introduced earlier as defining this book's underlying purpose: *Is any CAM therapy more effective than a placebo?* As a first step toward weighing that evidence, another question must be addressed: *What exactly is a placebo?*

CHAPTER TWO

A Brief History of Placebos

As far as we know, the first official use of the term "placebo" in a medical context occurred in a medical dictionary published in 1785, which defined a placebo therapy as something "calculated to amuse for a time."[1] Similarly, an 1811 definition characterized a placebo as something "given more to please than to benefit the patient."[2] Indeed, the Latin word *placebo* is commonly translated as "to please."

On the other hand, Patrick Wall, a well-known pain expert, argues that the medical use of this term may derive from the Latin version of Psalm 116:9, "Placebo Domino in regione vivorum," which in translation means "I will walk before the Lord in the land of the living." Wall hypothesizes that "placebo" later became a derogatory term to describe the work of priests and friars who were constantly badgering the populace for money to sing vespers for the dead—a speculation buttressed in the seventeenth century by Francis Bacon, a giant in the history of science, who used the term ironically: "instead of giving Free Counsel sing him song of placebo."[3]

While there is anecdotal evidence that some ancient physicians recognized the uniquely beneficial effects of a positive, authoritative presentation of a treatment regimen, we know for sure that nineteenth- and twentieth-century physicians increasingly became aware of a surprising phenomenon. When there was nothing that could be done for a specific complaint, these physicians sometimes prescribed what they knew were nonsensical therapies simply because they had found that the very act of prescribing *something* actually appeared to help their patients.

In some ways this is not particularly surprising, since prior to the twentieth century's refinements in analgesia (which greatly reduced the mortality rate from the crude surgical procedures previously available) and antibiotics (which, with the exception of vaccines, have probably saved more lives than all other medical innovations combined), relatively few effective pharmacologic therapies existed and major surgery was so traumatic that it was customarily used only as a last resort. In fact, some therapies (such as bloodletting) were so harmful that *any* noninvasive therapy without serious side effects must have been considered a medical boon by patients and practitioners alike. Even as late as the 1950s and early 1960s it was not uncommon for hospital pharmacies to stock both placebo pills (sugar) and injections (saline)—conveniently available in selected colors.

THE USE OF PLACEBOS IN RESEARCH

With a few notable exceptions to be described later in this chapter, the placebo effect itself escaped serious scientific scrutiny until 1955, having largely been considered prior to that time to be more a part of medical lore (or physician mystique) than a documented clinical entity. In that year, Dr. Henry K. Beecher published an article in the *Journal of the American Medical Association* titled "The Powerful Placebo" and, in the process, moved the placebo effect from the realm of myth into mainstream science.[4]

Beecher's research was relatively simple. He reanalyzed the results of fifteen clinical trials that had employed a placebo control group and concluded that 35 percent of the patients who had received a placebo responded positively. The article became an instant classic, and while a number of scientists have justifiably taken issue with his methods, Beecher's study proved quite influential in changing medical research practices because of the logical question it raised:

If patients participating in a clinical trial can improve simply because they believe *they are receiving an effective medical intervention, how can anyone have any confidence in the results of any clinical trial that did not employ a placebo control group?*

Taken to its logical extreme, this single finding implies that any nonharmful therapy evaluated by a trial without a placebo control group has the potential to produce positive results due to the placebo effect. In fact, even trials that employ other types of control groups (such as routine medical care) would also be suspect because the new therapy (effective or not) will produce a placebo effect, while patients who know they aren't receiving this innovative therapy will not have the benefit of a placebo effect.

For Beecher, the solution was patently clear: when a clinical trial is being conducted, patients must not be allowed to know whether or not they are receiving the experimental therapy. And since physicians are experts in producing placebo effects by carefully engendering positive expectations in their patients, it is important not to let them know, either.

The most effective way to avoid letting these cats out of their bags, Beecher reasoned, is to employ placebo control groups and to allow neither patients nor their providers to know who receives the experimental therapy and who receives the placebo therapy. Called "double blinding," this strategy soon became a scientific requirement for serious clinical trials and has since been employed for almost all types of medical interventions. Of course, creating credible placebo control groups is a lot easier in investigations of drug interventions (since a placebo capsule can be manufactured that is indistinguishable in taste, smell, and appearance from the active drug under evaluation) than is the case for other types of therapy. Still, though it is more difficult to guarantee the credibility of nonpharmaceutical placebos, these have now been successfully employed in everything from surgery (where a sham incision is performed under anesthesia) to acupuncture (where pointless needles appear to be inserted, or real needles are inserted in irrelevant locations).

It is almost solely within the scientific experimental arena, in fact, that the placebo effect possesses any importance in modern medicine. By comparison, the active use of placebos in patient care has declined, which may be partly due to a medical ethicist named Sissela Bok who, not long after Beecher's study, published an almost equally influential article in *Scientific American* titled "The Ethics of Giving Placebos."[5] Bok's conclusion was that their use in clinical practice was indeed unethical, and so today few if any hospital pharmacies stock placebo pills for anything other than their clinical trials.

Just because physicians no longer have sugar pills in their medicine cabinets, however, does not mean that they do not freely take advantage of the placebo effect in their day-to-day practices. A recent article in a peer-reviewed journal that I have edited for thirty years indicates that 86 percent of Danish general practitioners admitted they had employed a placebo treatment at least once during the past year, and 48 percent had used them ten times or more.[6] The most common uses (and remember, the practitioners wrote prescriptions or recommended these therapies knowing full well that they would have no effect on the conditions for which they were prescribed) were:

1. Antibiotics for viral infections
2. Physiotherapy
3. Sedatives for conditions other than depression
4. B vitamins for conditions such as multiple sclerosis and hair loss
5. Saline injections

There is little question, though, that the use of placebos as a treatment option has definitely fallen from favor in the United States over the past several decades. It is primarily to research specifically targeting the placebo effect, therefore, that we owe much of our rapidly growing knowledge about this effect and the conditions under which it occurs.

Undoubtedly a considerable amount of the impetus for this work can be attributed to Henry Beecher, because in science once a technique has been developed for reliably measuring something, it is as sure as death and taxes that that phenomenon will be the subject of further inquiry—and the placebo effect is no exception. There have been a plethora of studies performed on the phenomenon since Beecher's time, most of which have been designed to directly investigate the conditions under which the effect occurs, the methods by which the effect can be magnified, and the physiological mechanisms of action within the body that cause the set of reactions that we call placebo effects.

Ironically, in science, an almost universal result of conducting research important enough to encourage more work in the same area of inquiry is that the initial investigators will later be proved wrong, whether the subject matter is the placebo effect or quantum mechanics. It is even said that the ultimate compliment that any scientist can receive is to have done work that is important enough to encourage someone else to attack it.

By this standard, Henry Beecher's work was indeed important. Reanalyses of his methods and conclusions have demonstrated that his landmark study was so flawed that it did very little to actually establish the existence of the placebo effect, much less its proposed 35 percent effect size.[7] One reason for this failing is the still relatively common misconception that any gains or improvements observed by a placebo control group represent nothing but a placebo effect. Instead, what such gains represent are the effects of that entire class of logical and psychological impediments to logical thought that I alluded to earlier. True, the placebo is a prominent member of this community, but so too are artifacts such as the natural history of a disease (that is, the tendency for people to get better or worse during the course of an illness irrespective of any treatment at all), the fact that people behave differently when they are participating in an experiment than when they are not, a desire to please the experimental staff by providing socially desirable answers, and numerous other villains that I will discuss in detail later. What this means from a research perspective, therefore, is that as a general rule patients enrolled in clinical trials will witness some improvement over time regardless of whether the therapy being investigated works or not.

What Beecher apparently did not understand was that the only way to prove the existence of a placebo effect and to measure its size (at least in research designed to measure the effectiveness of a medical therapy) is to employ two control groups in the same experiment: one in which participants receive a placebo and one in which they receive no treatment at all.

While this is a relatively rare strategy, it is occasionally used, and the science of systematically locating such trials (and reanalyzing their combined results) has come a long way since Henry Beecher's time. Some years ago two Danish researchers (one of whom, Asbjorn Hrobjartsson, published the survey that I just discussed) were able to locate 114 clinical trials in which both types of controls were employed in the same study.[8] The authors, reporting their results in the *New England Journal of Medicine,* concluded that they had found "little evidence in general that placebos had powerful clinical effects" except for one notable exception: pain relief. Here, in the twenty-seven trials that involved this outcome (and encompassing a total of 1,602 patients), Hrobjartsson and Peter Gotzsche found that the difference between patients receiving no treatment at all and those receiving a placebo was indeed statistically significant in favor of the patients receiving placebos—hence confirming Beecher's original contention (at least for pain) by employing a considerably more rigorous methodology. (I like to think that this finding supplies a happy footnote to Beecher's distinguished scientific career. His research was important enough to generate more work, and the results of this work yielded the almost unprecedented benign judgment that his conclusions were largely correct—just for the wrong reasons.)

As is common practice in this field, Hrobjartsson and Gotzsche's conclusions were almost immediately attacked on the basis that they had underestimated the potency of the placebo effect by ignoring some studies with controls that actually offered some substantive form of treatment rather than no treatment at all.[9] All this ironically gives some credence to the conclusion reached by another set of researchers, Gunver Kienle and Helmut Kiene: "The placebo topic seems to invite sloppy methodological thinking."[10] But let's not quibble. While there is some excellent additional research suggesting that placebos can influence a number of conditions other than pain (such as depression, which—like pain—just happens to be measured by self-reports), the evidence is as close to incontrovertible for pain as we customarily get in science.

TOWARD A DEFINITION

Before we go any further, let's return for a moment to the question of definitions and look now at how modern scholars tend to define the placebo phenomenon. While not a fan of definitions for definitions' sake, I do believe that in this case they can highlight some very important characteristics of what a placebo effect is (and isn't)—not to mention the conditions necessary for one to manifest itself.

To understand the most commonly used definition of a placebo, it is helpful to recall that the primary use of placebos in modern medicine is for research purposes, where participants are randomly assigned to receive either an experimental drug or an identical-appearing inactive substance (placebo). This perspective, then, led to the following definition of a placebo:

> Any therapy or component of therapy (or that component of any therapy) that is intentionally or knowingly used for its non-specific, psychological, or psychophysiological effect, or for its presumed therapeutic effect on a patient, symptom, or other illness but is without specific activity for the condition being treated.[11]

While this is certainly a mouthful, the key notions here are of specific and nonspecific effects. A specific effect refers to the situation in which a drug contains a unique chemical substance that causes a biochemical reaction within the body that will cure a disease or relieve its symptoms.

Said another way, some other random chemical (or sugar pill) could not be substituted to produce the same effect. If indeed this were not the case, then the effect produced would be nonspecific.

Personally I find this definition a bit academic, but it does contain an important disclaimer: "or for its presumed therapeutic effect." This phrase is important because we usually assume there is some level of conscious deception involved in the administration of a placebo. This does not have to be the case, however, and we should keep this fact in mind when considering the types of placebo effects that occur in CAM. Many, if not most, CAM therapists are probably oblivious to the possibility that their elaborate machinations may in effect be engendering a placebo effect and nothing else.

Of course, if placebo effects could only be elicited consciously, placebo groups would not be necessary when conducting a randomized clinical trial. Honest scientists never set out to elicit only a placebo effect when they develop a new therapy. It is the realization that they can't avoid doing so that requires researchers to compensate for this totally natural phenomenon by randomly assigning half of their study participants to receive an inert placebo in the hope that their experimental drug will have a specific benefit over and above this nonspecific nuisance.

Now let me present a couple of definitions that I prefer:

A placebo effect is any genuine psychological or physiological response to an inert or irrelevant substance or procedure.[12]

And perhaps a bit more instructive for our purposes here:

A placebo is a pharmacologically inactive substance that can have a therapeutic effect if administered to a patient who believes that he or she is receiving an effective treatment.[13]

There are two key phrases here. The first, "a pharmacologically inactive substance," refers to the proverbial sugar pill containing no chemical substance that, by itself, is capable of curing a disease or reducing its symptoms. (One could substitute "a physiologically inactive procedure" in this definition to cover CAM therapies such as acupuncture.) The second key phrase, "if administered to a patient who believes that he or she is receiving an effective treatment," is what I like most about this definition. The phrase succinctly specifies the condition that must always accompany the pharmacologically inactive substance or procedure in order for a placebo effect to occur. In fact, it is this accompanying condition, the psychological state of belief (or expectation of benefit) on the part of the patient, that constitutes the crucial placebo component because, quite simply:

If the patient does not believe that he or she is receiving (or may be receiving) a potentially effective treatment, then no placebo effect will occur.

This is not true of a pharmacologically active substance. An antibiotic will cure bacterial infections whether the patient believes it will or not. It will even do so if it is administered when the patient is unconscious. A placebo, however, will have no effect on anything if the patient does not believe it will, and it most certainly will have no effect if it is administered while the patient is unconscious. In fact, perhaps a reasonable definition of a placebo would be:

Any medical treatment that can have a therapeutic effect only if administered to a patient who is aware that he or she is receiving a medical treatment.

But since most patients aren't unconscious (or suffering from dementia), allow me to end with one final, succinct definition for which I believe we've laid the foundation (and which, by the time everything is said and done, may wind up being the most applicable of all). This one was provided in an 1894 medical dictionary: "a make-believe medication."[14] Which could be amended to "a make-believe therapy."

THE EARLY USE OF PLACEBOS IN CAM RESEARCH

Ironically, one of the first recorded uses of a placebo for research purposes actually involved the evaluation of a CAM therapy more than two centuries ago. The therapy itself was the brainchild of an eighteenth-century Austrian physician named Franz Anton Mesmer, whose seminal contribution to science was the discovery that a combination of magnetic therapy and hypnotic suggestion was able to cure a wide range of patients suffering from an even wider range of maladies. Mesmer's theory regarding how the therapy worked involved a previously unrecognized natural energy source, similar to gravitation but more organic, hence termed "animal magnetism" by its discoverer. (It is fortunate that he did not name this energy after himself, since his name was later immortalized far more securely as a common-usage verb: "mesmerize.")

In a little-known historical footnote, and undoubtedly because of his professional interest in magnetism and electricity as well as his deserved rock-star-like intellectual celebrity in Europe, Benjamin Franklin became the principal investigator of a series of experiments designed to investigate Mesmer's new therapy. In describing the study itself, I borrow heavily from a colleague at Harvard, Ted J. Kaptchuk, who wrote a fascinating article that referenced the original 1785 description of this experiment.[15]

Franklin's involvement in these studies coincided with his crucial ambassadorship to France during the birth of his nation, but their historical relevance to the present issue is the fact that these experiments were among the first ever recorded in which a therapy (CAM or otherwise) was compared to a placebo. The process began by obtaining the help of a cooperating "mesmerist," who in turn identified a group of women who were known to be especially receptive to the therapy. First, these women were permitted to observe the mesmerist directing the energy toward them, after which they all reported being able to "feel" the energy in the body part to which it was directed. Next they were blindfolded (hence terms such as "blinded" and "double-blind" currently used in randomized, controlled trials) and asked if they could "feel" the energy.

Sure enough, they could. The trouble was, however, that when asked to identify the body part to which this energy was directed, they almost always identified the wrong part. Just to make sure that something really was amiss here, other experiments were conducted in which the mesmerist was placed in an adjacent room behind a screen and his energy was directed toward some subjects and not others. All the women were told that this new form of energy was being directed at them, and all of the women were able to "feel" the energy, regardless of whether it was actually directed at them or toward someone else.

The final experiment involved a young boy who had achieved some minor celebrity at the time by being especially sensitive to this new energy source. In Kaptchuk's words:

> A twelve-year-old boy subject, selected by the mesmerist, was led up to five trees, one of which had been mesmerized in Franklin's garden. Previously, the boy had routinely fainted in the presence of a mesmerized tree. This time he had his eyes covered with bandages so that there would be "no communication" between him and the mesmerist; he passed out and needed to be carried out of the garden when he embraced the wrong tree.[16]

None of this proved that mesmerists were all frauds or that their patients were willing partners in the deceptions involved. On the contrary, it is hard to imagine why either group would have subjected themselves to these procedures if they had not truly *believed* in the validity of what they were doing.

Instead, I prefer to interpret these experiments, more than 200 years old, as demonstrations of how susceptible both patients *and* practitioners are to allowing their expectations (and the suggestions of others) to cloud their judgment, how closely intertwined CAM therapeutic and placebo effects have been historically, and how important it is to employ placebo controls in experiments designed to investigate modern-day CAM therapies. And if you feel some tinge of pity for poor Mesmer's place in history, don't. He is the proud father of a well-respected present-day CAM therapy: hypnotism (whose advocates seldom mention his original discrediting).

RELEVANCE TO AN IMPORTANT
SCIENTIFIC PRINCIPLE

Perhaps in recognition of this historical and conceptual similarity between CAM therapies and placebos, the National Center for Complementary and Alternative Medicine now actually funds research into the placebo effect itself. It is also justifiably loath to fund any clinical trial that does not incorporate some mechanism to control for it.[17] Why? Because the simple acts of enrolling people in a scientific experiment and providing them with a therapy that they believe has the potential of being effective will indeed result in these individuals feeling that they have been helped. Hence, guided by Benjamin Franklin and all of the other NIH institutes' example, the National Center for Complementary and Alternative Medicine now requires that some effort be expended to keep patients from knowing whether they are receiving a "real" CAM therapy or a "fake" one.

This is a crucial requirement because CAM therapies share something important with placebos: both are typically administered only in the presence of an expectation of benefit, whether this takes place in a research setting or in a practitioner's office. But what if CAM therapies and placebos were also found to have something else in common—namely, the same documented effects upon subjective outcomes such as pain and psychological affect—but neither was actually capable of curing anything? If indeed all of this turned out to be true, and if common sense counted for anything, then perhaps we might conclude that two things producing the same results for the same reasons and always requiring the same conditions to occur in the first place might just be the *same thing*. Or, in the words of a truly great scientific philosopher whose name escapes me:

If something looks like a duck and quacks like a duck, then it probably is a duck.

On the other hand, if there is high-quality, scientific evidence that placebos and CAM therapies do not share all of these characteristics, then most likely they aren't one and the same thing. It is this very evidence that will be considered later in this book. First, however, it is important for us to examine the nature of scientific evidence itself and to understand especially how it can be corrupted by that extended family I've mentioned several times before—that is, the family of logical, psychological, and physiological impediments to connecting cause and effect that necessitates the conduct of scientific research in the first place. These are equal-opportunity impediments, incidentally, that operate to confound us all: scientists, patients, and physicians.

CHAPTER THREE

Natural Impediments to Making Valid Inferences

There are a lot of people out there who believe that they are being helped by CAM therapies. There are even a lot of people who believe that diluted cuttlefish discharge has potent curative powers. So if there are tens of millions of people in the United States alone (and probably hundreds of millions worldwide) who have used CAM therapies and believe them to be effective, why consider what science has to say about this issue? Framed from a slightly different perspective: if the majority of the human race (along with generations of their grandparents) believes that therapies such as acupuncture, chiropractic manipulation, and homeopathy can relieve pain and cure disease, would anyone questioning such a judgment also have to question the intelligence of his species?

The answer is definitely no. Instead, we should question what influences our thought processes. To decide whether something is effective or not requires us to engage in an extremely complex (and quintessentially human) activity involving the *generation of correct causal inferences*. And this is exactly what we automatically and unconsciously do every time we visit a health practitioner of any sort (or self-medicate ourselves, or place crystals in the window, or wear magnets or ionized bracelets) to achieve relief from noxious symptoms.

In other words, if our knee hurts and we go to an acupuncturist who places small needles in our leg, we ask ourselves questions such as:

Did my knee stop hurting (or hurt less) after the needles were inserted?

Did my knee stop hurting (or hurt less) in the days and weeks following the needle insertion?

If the answer to either of these questions is yes, we ask ourselves (again usually automatically and subconsciously):

Did my knee stop hurting (or hurt less) *because* of what the acupuncturist did?

Arriving at a correct answer to this third question is a very difficult task given our propensity to make incorrect assumptions in the absence of some very relevant information that we often don't even recognize we need to know in the first place. And this difficulty is further compounded in the presence of something like a placebo effect that—unrecognized—actually conspires to provide us with misinformation.

So no, people don't make mistakes in arriving at causal inferences because they are stupid. They make them because of very real impediments that initially give rise to belief in things such as CAM and visits by extraterrestrials. It is, in fact, the existence of such impediments to making correct causal inferences that necessitated one of our species' greatest achievements: the scientific process.

CAUSAL INFERENCES

The types of inference with which we are concerned in this book revolve around reaching a conclusion that the occurrence of a phenomenon (pain relief) was caused by the introduction of something that preceded it (a CAM therapy) and *nothing* else. This would appear to be a very straightforward conclusion, unless there were such things as placebos lurking in the background that were capable of producing the same phenomenon (or unless this phenomenon, pain reduction, would have occurred even if the patient had not visited his or her CAM therapist). Then this type of inference becomes much more difficult to make and the conclusion that the CAM therapy caused the symptom relief becomes much more tenuous.

Most people probably couldn't care less what the real cause was as long as they did experience a reduced level of pain. However, if the pain eventually comes back—and it inevitably will return if it is caused by a chronic condition—then the patient will be forced to go to the CAM therapist again (or change the location of the magnets). Even then, it is quite possible that the same sort of extraneous factors (of which the placebo effect is only one example) may continue to operate, reinforcing the patient's original inferential error. This process may continue for many visits and perhaps even for many years, thus ensuring the survival of the therapy and the continued income of the therapist. True, some patients may eventually realize that the therapy does not really work or, more likely, that the therapy no longer works for them, but by then their word of mouth has contributed to the support of both the therapist and the therapy.

Scientists and physicians, on the other hand, do care whether or not CAM therapies actually cause a reduction in people's symptoms or actually cure their diseases. Physicians care because they need to know whether these CAM therapies should be prescribed in lieu of, or in addition to, the treatments they currently employ. This is their job, after all: to help all of their patients—even those who haven't tried CAM. Scientists care because they need to *understand* things, which means that ultimately they need to know the true causes and effects of everything.

But why should nonscientists care one iota about something as esoteric as a causal inference? I believe that the answer to this question is because the making of causal inferences is part of our job description as *Homo sapiens*. Undoubtedly it was a historical condition for our survival as a species as well. Or, as Michael Shermer more eloquently puts it, we by necessity "evolved to be skilled, pattern-seeking, causal-finding creatures. Those who were best at finding patterns (standing upwind of game animals is bad for the hunt, cow manure is good for the crops) left behind the most offspring. We are their descendents."[1]

So let's examine what is involved in this pattern-seeking search for understanding. On their most simplistic level, causal inferences are synonymous with the ability to connect consequences with actions: Y follows X, therefore Y was caused by X. On their most complex level, causal inferences are synonymous with answering questions that begin with *why*. On their most pragmatic level, they constitute the mechanism by which we experiment with things in our everyday lives to find what is good for us and what is not. We do this by observing what happens following our little experiments and then by deciding whether or not these outcomes were produced by the specific actions we were implementing. Most people don't conceptualize their lives this way, but all of us are inveterate scientists and experimenters. We constantly conduct experiments on ourselves (or our social and physical environments do it for us), and although we don't think of them as scientific, their results are often more important to us personally than anything appearing in a scientific journal.

Unfortunately, patterns (to use Michael Shermer's language), especially causal ones, are often extremely difficult to recognize, partly because they are hard to differentiate from simple coincidences. And even when they are recognized, the inferential leap to a valid, causal inference is much more tenuous than most people realize.

Like everything else, some causal inferences are simpler than others. When the consequence immediately and inevitably follows the action, our brains, like those of most mammals, can very quickly infer that the action is the cause of the consequence and learn to either perform or avoid the indicated action. A child, for example, needs only one lesson to learn that touching a stove's reddened electric coil or a campfire's open flame will immediately and inevitably result in a painful burn.

Other causal inferences can be considerably more difficult to make, even though they may eventually seem obvious, given our ability to communicate our discoveries to one another. As an example, consider one of the consequences of having sex—pregnancy. If two primitive individuals had sex, the woman might or might not become pregnant. Even if she did, she would not know about the pregnancy for several months after the sexual encounter. She would therefore be much more likely to attribute her condition to some completely extraneous event that immediately preceded her first awareness of her condition than to connect it to a sexual encounter that occurred several months earlier. Perhaps her pregnancy would be attributed to an herb she had recently developed a taste for. Perhaps it would be because she had wanted a child and had persuaded her mate to give a fresh kill to a local shaman. Or perhaps the interruption in her menstrual cycle would be interpreted as the true cause of her pregnancy. Of course, the more pregnancies the couple experienced, the more likely they would be to connect the proper action with this consequence, but there would be no guarantee that they would ever make the connection.

If our couple were part of a social group that verbally communicated with one another, however, the connection between sexual intercourse and pregnancy would eventually be recognized by someone (who thousands of years later would have been called a scientist) based upon the available data, and this discovery would be passed down orally to other generations—perhaps first emanating from the observation of domestic animals, where the actions and consequences occur closer together and the link between them is more easily observed. We don't know how long such word-of-mouth processes took, but the best guess is a very long time indeed. (We also know that *incorrect* causal inferences are made and passed on the same way, although presumably they don't take as long to formulate.)

Seven conditions can make this type of inference very difficult:

1. The consequence does not inevitably occur as a result of the action (sexual intercourse).
2. The consequence does not appear immediately.
3. The consequence is not intuitively connected with the action.
4. The consequence can occur in the absence of any action on the part of its recipient whatever.

5. The consequence can occur as a result of any number of other actions.
6. The consequence is not absolute but rather is measured in terms of a subtle gradient.
7. The component has a large subjective component (and hence may be real or imagined).

Inferences made under the last four conditions are notoriously unreliable, not because people are unobservant but because so many extraneous events can occur between the action and the consequence that it becomes more likely than not that an irrelevant event will be selected as the true cause. To illustrate, let us consider a concrete example of these extremely difficult causal inferences in light of the aforementioned seven disconnects.

Let's begin with someone suffering persistent pain in, say, the left knee. The pain has lasted longer than its recipient believes that it should. Let's further assume that this person's primary care physician prescribed a nonsteroidal anti-inflammatory drug that provided some temporary relief but eventually resulted in stomach discomfort worse than the original knee pain.

This, dear reader, is really where our story begins. For at some point in our history we, as humans, began adapting our environment to our own needs rather than the other way around, to the extent that it is now against our nature to accept our fate without a struggle—which in turn means that we as a species have become inveterate experimenters. In other words, we are all scientists. We have to be. If a serious problem arises, it is written in our genes that we must try to solve it.

Thus what does our patient do? Simply live with the pain? No, at least not at first, and probably not until after he has searched for other possible ways to stop the pain. He may go back to his doctor. He may call his grandmother or a friend and ask what that person did for knee pain. He may go online and comb through the countless sites that address knee pain and make claims about what to do about it: exercise, cold packs, physical therapy, acupuncture, and so on. Let's say that for one reason or another our patient opts to try acupuncture and after a few sessions discovers that the pain has begun to dissipate.

At first glance, figuring out whether or not the acupuncture was responsible for relieving this individual's pain would appear to be a no-brainer. In truth, however, it requires linking a consequence (pain relief) to an action (acupuncture) that is potentially disconnected at all seven of the aforementioned points and is therefore subject to a wide range of inferential impediments that must somehow be overcome. Let us examine each of these disconnects in a bit more detail before going on to the attendant artifacts that make them so difficult to bridge:

- **Points 1 and 2:** *The consequence (pain relief) does not inevitably follow the action, or if it does, it doesn't always occur immediately.* Even a truly effective therapy often takes some time to work. So if queried ahead of time, few experienced (or savvy) acupuncturists would claim that their therapy *always,* under *all* circumstances, reduces their clients' pain. Sometimes, they will say, the pain is too intense, or the patient is too preoccupied (or stressed), or something prevented the elicitation of the full effect. Or sometimes they will say that the effects are cumulative or are inexplicably delayed for a period of time. All of these claims could be true, or they might just be another way of explaining spontaneous remission.

- **Point 3:** *The real cause is counterintuitive.* The logical fallacy *post hoc, ergo propter hoc* (after this, therefore because of this) is so ingrained in all of us that it would be very difficult for our hypothetical patient to believe that his acupuncture sessions just happened to coincide with, say, the natural cessation of the unpleasant symptoms. And it would probably be even more difficult to imagine that the simple *expectation* of pain relief (that is, the placebo effect) could result in something being released by the brain that could actually *result* in pain relief.

- **Point 4:** *The consequence can occur in the absence of any known action.* This is the greatest impediment that confronts us in evaluating the effectiveness of something such as a CAM therapy, more problematic even than the placebo effect or any of the members of its extended family. When we do nothing at all, the vast majority of the unpleasant symptoms that occur in our daily lives disappear on their own due to the body's ability to eventually heal itself. Often this process takes longer than we would like and we get discouraged, pessimistically assuming that the symptoms are truly chronic and will never go away without a magic bullet of some sort. But in most cases we do get better. (Physicians like to call this spontaneous remission.) Hence if our hypothetical patient were in this situation and stuck with acupuncture long enough, it's likely that he would eventually be "cured"—not by acupuncture but simply by the body's built-in mechanisms. Alternatively, if a succession of CAM therapies were tried, *one* of them would by necessity eventually coincide with this remissive process. Hence that CAM therapy would be judged to have "worked," and there is no way that anyone anywhere would ever convince our happy patient that it might be something other than the CAM therapy itself that wrought this magic.

- **Point 5:** *The consequence can occur as a result of a number of alternative actions.* In our pregnancy example, there is only one way to get pregnant (at least in a low-tech world), but pain can dissipate in many, many ways—including as a result of the person being distracted by something else, of some other lifestyle change, or of completely unknown causes.

- **Points 6 and 7:** *The consequence is subjectively measured on a gradient and is very difficult to verify independently.* Only someone suffering from pain can validly report its presence and intensity. These subjective reports of pain (or other unpleasant symptoms) are far less precise than laboratory results, due in part to several facts: (1) they are not all-or-nothing propositions but rather are sometimes more extreme and sometimes less, (2) there are large individual (and even cultural) differences in symptom tolerance, (3) symptoms tend to be multifaceted, with many different manifestations (pain, for example, can be throbbing, stinging, burning and so forth), (4) our perceptions of symptoms can be masked or accentuated by other conditions (e.g., pain in another part of the body, stress, anxiety, or even how preoccupied we are by the tasks we are performing), (5) sometimes our symptoms aren't even "real"—that is, biologically defined—but are completely psychosomatic, and (6) once our symptoms dissipate our memories of their intensity are notoriously unreliable. So it follows that any causal inferences based upon these imprecise sensory signals must by necessity possess a degree of imprecision themselves.

Thus while each of these disconnects is problematic enough in its own right, they are especially deleterious when combined with an entire family of omnipresent logical, statistical, and psychological impediments to our inferential abilities. Such artifacts are as much a part of our human environment as the air we breathe.

What I would like to do in the remainder of this chapter, then, is to begin to delve into the difficulties of making causal inference when these artifacts are allowed to operate unchecked. To facilitate this process, allow me to employ a case study: the experiences of my late mother-in-law.

SARAH'S STORY

During the latter part of her eighty-five-year life, Sarah Cohen, an intelligent, still very sharp former concert pianist, began, like most people her age, to experience a number of unpleasant symptoms often involving pain. At first she took her complaints to her internist, who would dutifully prescribe something that might or might not work.

Then she began to realize that her internist had a very limited repertoire of options and an even more limited amount of time available to hear her complaints (complaints, incidentally, which her physician knew were not life-threatening and which he judged to be simply part of the aging process). So, being an independent, take-charge sort of individual, she subscribed to *Prevention* magazine in order to learn more about the multiple remedies suggested in each month's issue for symptoms such as those she was experiencing. For anyone not familiar with *Prevention,* it sometimes bills itself as the "largest health magazine [in terms of sales] in the world," but as its owner and my former patron, Robert Rodale, used to be fond of saying, it is really a magazine more about *self-care* than about prevention. It was (and is) also very much about CAM, although this term had not been coined before Rodale's untimely death in a car accident.

Then things changed for Sarah and she was afflicted by pain in one of her knees that didn't ever seem to go away and that her internist (who didn't experience the pain) diagnosed as a mild case of osteoarthritis of the knee. At his suggestion, Sarah saw a rheumatologist, who confirmed the internist's diagnosis, wrote her a prescription for a pain medication (probably accompanied by instructions that she take the medication twice a day or as needed), and suggested that she make a return appointment three months later. History has not recorded whether she kept the appointment, but we can infer that Sarah (like almost 100 percent of arthritis sufferers) was not completely satisfied with her treatment—either because of frequent side effects or because of the unfortunate fact that it provided only partial, temporary relief for her pain.

One thing that Sarah's Boswell can record with assurance, however, was that every couple of months she would breathlessly give her daughter and your author a call and announce with great enthusiasm and conviction that she had just started this or that food supplement or nutraceutical recommended in *Prevention* magazine and that it had practically cured her arthritis. While this was certainly perceived by us as most excellent news, we did begin to notice that she never made mention of the previous miracle cure over which she had waxed so enthusiastic just a few months earlier.

Now, it should be mentioned that Sarah was not given to gullibility. In fact, if anything, she might be described as overly suspicious— perhaps forgivable in someone who spent her youth hiding from the Nazis in Belgium while her family in Poland was being obliterated. What, then, was going on with Sarah's thought processes? Assuming that she did not have a serious memory deficit (which she almost certainly did not, since she could still play dozens of major pieces without access to sheet music) or reasoning deficiency (which she definitely did not, since she considered your author one of the greatest sons-in-law, husbands, and fathers of all time), what was it that was conspiring to induce Sarah to make so many false positive inferences?

The answer is multilayered but not complex. A number of logical and psychological impediments to logical inference (including but not limited to the placebo effect) were conspiring to trick her into believing in the effectiveness of these basically bogus therapies. Here's how the process might have played out for Sarah.

The Natural History of Pain

Like most arthritis sufferers, Sarah's pain waxed and waned with time. She had some periods of extreme discomfort, some periods where it was bothersome but tolerable enough that she felt no need for medication, and even some days when she scarcely felt any pain at all.

Let's pretend that the graph in Figure 3.1 is a simplified representation of Sarah's normal knee pain when absolutely nothing was done for it. The metric (which runs from 0 to 10) represented by the vertical line to the left is called a visual analog scale and is, in many research and clinical settings, the preferred way to quantify how much pain someone is suffering (Figure 3.2).[2] The technique consists of a simple line containing eleven hash marks ranging from 0 ("no pain at all") to 10 ("severe pain" or "intolerable pain"). The patient (or research participant) is asked to place a mark on the line representing how much pain he or she is experiencing

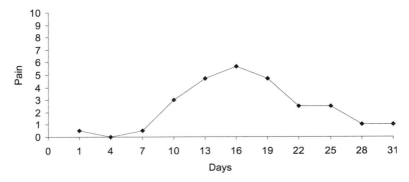

Figure 3.1. Hypothetical Natural History of Sarah's Arthritis Pain

at the time of the assessment or, say, on average has experienced during the past twenty-four hours. As simplistic as this technique seems, it is about as valid a way as we have to measure pain, since no one but the individual experiencing pain can reliably quantify it.

But let's return to the thirty-one-day graph of Sarah's knee pain (Figure 3.1). Since Sarah did not have an advanced case of arthritis (and since arthritis is a chronic rather than acute condition), her pain never reached as high as the 7 mark and actually hit zero once during the month. Now, remembering that this graph represents completely un-treated pain in the absence of her rheumatologist's prescription or even some-over-the counter medications, consider the following question:

If Sarah decided to try some glucosamine tablets, which had been highly touted in her magazine, at what point in this curve would she be most likely to do so?

Certainly not at day 1, when her pain was almost nonexistent. Probably not day 22 either, when it seemed to be on the decline. The best guess would be around day 15, when her pain had reached a peak.

Now, just for argument's sake, let's pretend that glucosamine is completely worthless and does not work at all. In other words, let's assume that this particular CAM therapy contains no active ingredient

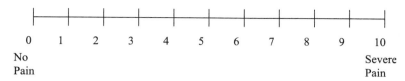

Figure 3.2. Visual Analog Scale Used in Pain Research

that is capable of affecting pain one iota. Let's also forsake our advantage of hindsight and pretend that neither we nor Sarah had access to any information at all regarding her normal pain cycle. Let's pretend instead that Sarah started recording her pain level on day 16 (right after she started her CAM treatment) and stopped doing so at day 31, after it appeared to have leveled off at a manageable level. Let's further assume that we were presented with these data (which are depicted in Figure 3.3) and asked to arrive at a conclusion as to whether or not we believed glucosamine worked.

Assuming normal eyesight, the answer should be obvious. As soon as Sarah started taking glucosamine, her pain began to subside. If we were to compare day 16 with day 31 (as many research studies do), how could we fail to conclude that glucosamine was indeed effective in reducing arthritis pain?

Unfortunately, this principle of *post hoc, ergo propter hoc*, which is extremely effective for simple causal relationships in which the consequence immediately and inevitably follows the action, is the primary cause of error when making complex causal inferences. It is also the mother of all superstitions—consider the basketball coach who happened to be wearing a red coat when the team won a crucial game and then feels compelled to keep wearing it until the team begins to lose.

But in Sarah's case, we know the truth ahead of time (which is a rare luxury in life and unheard of in science). We know from Figure 3.1 that her pain was going to subside anyway because we know what the natural history of her condition was. We also know (because of our earlier assumption) that glucosamine has no specific pain-dampening properties of its own. Naturally, however, Sarah wouldn't make such an

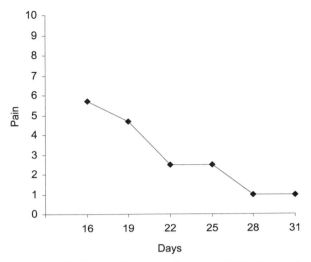

Figure 3.3. Natural History Masquerading as a CAM Analgesic Effect

assumption, and, being a sensible person, she would be expected to come to a different conclusion and to behave accordingly. She would keep taking her miracle cure, at least until it became clear to her that it wasn't the miracle for which she had been searching. But, as sure as day follows night, her pain would begin to peak in a few weeks and she would either immediately give up on her CAM therapy or suffer through a few more cycles. Eventually she would either consciously realize that the glucosamine was really doing her no good or unconsciously be more susceptible to looking favorably upon another of *Prevention* magazine's recommendations. And so the entire cycle would repeat itself.

But given Sarah's perspicacity, chances are that natural history alone, even coupled with her very real desire to live a normal, pain-free life, might not have been enough to have ensured her continuing these little personal experiments indefinitely—always characterized as they were by initial success followed by disappointment. Fortunately for *Prevention* magazine, the manufacturers of the nutraceuticals and food supplements that it touted, and perhaps even Sarah herself, there was something out there that did work quite reliably, and this something is probably the first medical treatment, conventional or CAM, ever discovered: the placebo.

The Placebo Effect's Role in Sarah's Experiments

If there were no such thing as a placebo effect, Sarah would probably have eventually recognized the rhythm of her pain, which she initially mistook as evidence of CAM's therapeutic "successes" (during days 16 through 31 in Figure 3.1, when her pain was declining naturally) or "failures" (days 4 through 16, when it was on the rise). Unlike the natural history of her disease, however, the placebo effect is not something that occurs "naturally." It must be *manufactured* in the sense that it occurs *only* in the presence of therapeutic intent (or the perception of such intent).

Could Sarah ever have suspected its presence? Certainly neither *Prevention* nor the companies that sold glucosamine would have mentioned it to her, since it was not in their best interest to do so and they probably believed in what they were selling anyway. Certainly her physician wouldn't have said anything to her about it either, because she didn't even tell him what she was doing for fear that he wouldn't approve (and because she was afraid that he would take it as an indirect indictment of the care he was giving her). Still, as the wife of a physician, Sarah would have heard about the placebo effect. Perhaps she never would have believed herself susceptible to such a "weakness" because she was rightly proud of her strong-mindedness and common sense. Surely she would have thought that she had nothing in common with people who are susceptible to something as transparent as the mere *suggestion* that a therapy might be beneficial.

But in truth, we are probably hardwired to be susceptible to both suggestion and conditioning because of their importance in facilitating learning, so in retrospect the occurrence of a placebo effect was probably inevitable in Sarah's case. From the opening bell, she enrolled herself in her one-woman trials for several reasons:

- She *believed* that the therapies she was trying would be (or at least could be) effective in reducing her pain. We can probably thank *Prevention* magazine for partially instilling this belief due to its persuasive articles, which reported not just anecdotal testimonials from other patients whose personal "clinical trials" had been victims of the same artifacts as Sarah's but also case studies supplied by clinicians who, as will be discussed in Chapter 4, are unwittingly exposed to even more of these false-positive-producing artifacts.

- She *hoped* that the therapy would work, based upon her past suffering.

- She *had been reinforced* by trying previous interventions recommended by her physician that had (at least initially) resulted in some improvement due to, among other things, natural history, the placebo effect, and perhaps even an honest-to-goodness active chemical ingredient in the medication itself.

In short, the main precursors for a full-blown dose of the placebo effect were in place: belief in the efficacy of the treatment, desire (or motivation) for relief, and classical conditioning.

And if all of this weren't pernicious enough, the placebo effect occurs independently of (thus in addition to) all of the other logical artifacts that affect our inferences. To illustrate, let's see how the placebo effect might interact with Sarah's natural history of pain depicted earlier.

The Placebo Effect Occurring During a Period of Intense Pain

First, let's examine what might have happened had Sarah begun her experiment somewhere near day 16, which was the zenith of her pain cycle. The solid line in Figure 3.4 represents the cyclical nature of Sarah's

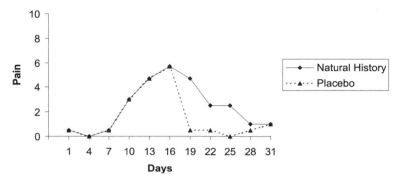

Figure 3.4. The Placebo Effect Added to a Natural History Effect

pain, showing the levels of pain that would have occurred had she not had the benefit of a placebo effect. The dotted line, on the other hand, illustrates what might have occurred when the placebo effect was introduced into this experiment.

In other words, Sarah's pain still decreases, but much more dramatically. Is it any wonder that such an effect would prompt so enthusiastic a call to her family?

The Placebo Effect Occurring During a Period of Increasing Pain

While Sarah might not have been able to identify the exact points at which her pain reached its zenith, she almost surely would have chosen an intervention point at which it was sufficiently troublesome to spur her into some kind of action. To illustrate, Figure 3.5 shows what would have happened had she chosen day 10 to take her first glucosamine capsule.

This particular timing of the glucosamine (placebo) would have probably produced an equally dramatic phone call if Sarah was unconsciously expecting her pain to continue to increase to something approximating day 16 (the solid line), as it had in the past. In other words, our experimenter might have concluded, correctly, that she had headed off a very unpleasant experience by taking her capsules. But it

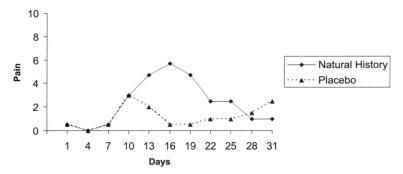

Figure 3.5. The Placebo Effect Occurring During a Period of Naturally Increasing Pain

was the *taking* of the capsules, not anything in them, that prevented the pain from increasing. In other words, she would have been correct for the wrong reason.

As a species, we are almost surely genetically programmed to draw causal conclusions, since the ability to draw correct (and often quick) ones was almost surely an important survival skill—resulting from (and/or contributing to) the evolution of our brain size. However, most of these early inferences probably involved consequences that immediately and inevitably followed a specific action. I would guess that the ability to recognize more abstract patterns developed later and was greatly facilitated by the increased sophistication of language and societal structures. Perhaps what spawned the development of the scientific process was actually the complexities involved in making inferences in which the consequences did not inevitably and immediately follow their actions, were capable of being caused by alternative actions, and involved actions that themselves had to be inferred rather than observed. (Perhaps this promulgated the development of religion as well, but that is a path upon which I prefer not to tread.)

The bottom line for us here is that the placebo effect, in conjunction with factors such as the natural history of our symptoms, conspires to produce false positive conclusions in the small, personal (but important) "clinical trials" that Sarah routinely conducted on herself. And while these particular hurdles are probably universal, there are a number of other impediments to causal thinking whose presence varies among individuals.

PSYCHOLOGICAL FACTORS IMPEDING OUR ABILITY TO DRAW CORRECT CAUSAL INFERENCES

In truth, there are a plethora of psychological, biochemical, statistical, and logical impediments that interfere with our ability to make complex inferences and that thereby conspire to produce false positive results in our little everyday experiments. While we can't consider them all, and while classifications such as physiological versus psychological are ultimately arbitrary, there are six thought patterns that I nevertheless think are especially relevant to our perceptions about CAM therapies:

- *A reluctance to admit when we are wrong (cognitive dissonance).*[3] In Sarah's case this might have begun when she read something extolling the virtues of a supplement that seemed plausible enough to have encouraged her to spend some of her retirement money to purchase it—perhaps even explicitly going against the advice of her physician or a trusted confidant in doing so. It therefore might have been quite difficult for her to have consciously admitted that she had been wrong, had wasted her money, and perhaps had been duped by someone—especially when she took such justifiable pride in her good judgment.

- *Simple optimism (possessing an internal locus of control).* This would take the form of Sarah believing, like Agent Mulder in *The X Files*, that there must be "something out there" that could control her pain without side effects. If this belief were strong enough, it could single-handedly predispose her to erroneously assign a positive result to her experiments.

- *Respect for authority.* This is the time-honored tendency for people to accept the word of individuals with special credentials, and it is quite capable of coloring our assessment of the consequences of following these individuals' recommendations. The fostering of this attribute is the reason some practitioners (both CAM and conventional) wear white coats and display their credentials on their walls.

- *A* National Enquirer *approach to life.* What I mean by this is our built-in propensity (or need) to believe the absurd. Some people, given the choice of a traditional scientific explanation versus the most ridiculous, counterintuitive rationale possible, appear to inevitably choose the latter. Whether this is due to a conscious choice, some kind of alternative worldview, or just a desire to believe in wondrous occurrences that are never seen in everyday life, I do not know.

- *A conspiracy-oriented view of the world.* This is related to the *National Enquirer* outlook but is more paranoid in nature and often explains the lack of scientific evidence to back one's beliefs about governmental or special interest cover-ups. This is exemplified by the belief, for example, that the government has been covering up abductions by aliens or the identities of the true assassins of John F. Kennedy for decades. In CAM it is epitomized by Kevin Trudeau, author of the best-selling book *Natural Cures "They" Don't Want You to Know About,* which reveals that the only reason his natural cures for just about every conceivable human ailment aren't in wider use is governmental and industry cover-ups.

- *A complete lack of skepticism.* This can be translated as either complete gullibility or (more charitably) trustfulness.

Regardless of how we classify them, all of these impediments to making complex causal inferences are capable of explaining why so many people could be so wrong about the effectiveness of things such as CAM therapies. And we haven't even considered the most important yet, for far and away the most potent contributor to these potentially incorrect inferences lies in the dynamics characterizing the patient-healer dyad. Unlike Sarah, most patients do not engage in CAM therapies in isolation, and it is the actual presence of a healer that provides the strongest known impetus for engendering a placebo effect. This is especially true for the healer who believes in what he or she does, who has the patient's best interests at heart, and in whose competence the patient believes. While every profession has unprincipled practitioners, I would hazard a guess that most CAM therapists believe fervently in the value of what they are doing. In fact, it may be that the most effective strategies available to any of these practitioners are these beliefs and the resultant placebo effects they engender.

But to be fair, it is not just CAM therapists who believe in CAM therapies. Many conventional physicians, while perhaps not allotting much credence to some of the biologically less plausible practices such as homeopathy or psychic healing, do believe that certain of the more invasive ones (most notably, acupuncture) can effectively reduce pain. Which leads to a question similar to the one that began this chapter:

If so many highly trained, compassionate clinicians—individuals numbering among the best and brightest members of our species—believe that CAM therapies are effective, why even consider what science has to say about the issue?

And of course the answer is the same as it was for the original question—involving the very same difficulties inherent in making correct causal inferences in the hostile epistemological environment called everyday life, plus a few new challenges that are unique to everyday clinical practice.

CHAPTER FOUR

Impediments That Prevent Physicians and Therapists from Making Valid Inferences

It's one thing to hypothesize how someone like Sarah can be tricked into believing that a CAM therapy is helping her when nothing is operating except placebo effects, the natural history of pain, and a few Psych 101 concepts such as cognitive dissonance. It's still another to explain how a highly trained, skilled, and compassionate physician can be tricked into believing a placebo is really a miraculous panacea. Here is one scenario demonstrating how such a state of affairs could come to pass.

DR. SMITH'S STORY

Unlike most people, Dr. Smith knew exactly what he wanted to do in life from the time he was in the eighth grade. He wanted to have a job in which he could eventually make a good living by actually helping people. He wanted, in other words, to be a physician, and he was willing to go to medical school for the privilege of working more than eighty hours a week for several years—first as a low-paid intern and then as a low-paid medical resident.

After clearing these considerable hurdles, and after establishing his own internal medicine practice (the latter accomplished before the ascent of managed care), he began to achieve his original goals: making a good living by helping people. And yet his practice, while satisfying, did hold one frustration that increasingly bothered him as the years passed: his inability to help patients like Sarah, who experienced chronic pain. True, analgesics often worked for a while, but they ultimately left a good deal to be desired.

So, in order to keep abreast of the latest medical developments in pain management, Dr. Smith joined the International Association for the Study of Pain (IASP), a society that publishes a peer-reviewed journal solely devoted to pain research, aptly named *Pain*. At the society's annual conference one year, Dr. Smith attended a number of presentations devoted to acupuncture research and was intrigued enough to join the society's acupuncture special interest group. From this special interest group's newsletter, he learned that there had been a considerable amount of research conducted to evaluate acupuncture's ability to reduce pain, and he was so impressed by its reports of the promising results of this research that he correspondingly used one of his precious summer vacations to attend a workshop designed to teach its participants the basic skills of acupuncture therapy.

Soon after his return he gave one of his oldest patients, Mrs. Jones, the option of receiving several acupuncture sessions in addition to the nonsteroidal anti-inflammatory drugs she normally used only when her arthritis pain was at its worst. Mrs. Jones accepted his invitation and, heartened by her clinical response, Dr. Smith tried it on several other patients, the majority of whom also showed marked improvement.

Dr. Smith soon became, based upon his clinical experiences, an avid advocate of acupuncture for almost all types of chronic pain and even published a paper in a medical journal based upon a case study involving one of his more interesting patients. While the genesis of his inference regarding the efficacy of acupuncture may appear obvious and unassailable, as do his motives for practicing it, a natural question arises:

*Could Dr. Smith's inference regarding the efficacy of acupuncture be
as flawed as Sarah's were concerning glucosamine?*

And if so:

What could have contributed to his erroneous conclusion?

The answer to the first question is yes, and the answer to the second
one is the usual suspects (plus a couple more unique to Dr. Smith's
situation).

SOME LOGICAL ARTIFACTS BEDEVILING CLINICAL INFERENCES

While Dr. Smith, like Sarah, would never conceptualize it this way, every
time he treated a patient (especially when he did so in a novel way or
when the patient arrived at his office with a novel condition), he was in
the process of conducting his very own small-scale experiment. To illustrate, let's return to Dr. Smith's first acupuncture patient, Mrs. Jones,
upon whom he had previously and unsuccessfully tried just about every
medication he could think of.

When she showed up at his office every month or so complaining that
her arthritis pain was "driving her crazy," Dr. Smith felt as if it was he who
was being driven crazy. For while he cared deeply about all of his patients,
Mrs. Jones had been with him the longest and occupied a special place in
his heart. Following the summer of his forfeited vacation, it was therefore
no accident that Mrs. Jones was the first patient he told about the acupuncture training he had just received. The therapy, he informed her, was
of ancient Chinese lineage, and one that a number of randomized clinical
trials had demonstrated to be of considerable help in reducing arthritis pain. Being an ethical individual, Dr. Smith informed his patient that
while there was no guarantee that it would work for her, he personally
believed that it might help her. He also may have informed her that it was

the only thing he could think of at this point that had any chance at all of doing so.

His patient, who knew he cared about her, was aware that he had her best interests at heart, and had a great deal of respect for his clinical judgment, readily agreed. What neither of them realized was that they had just designed one of the most biased, completely uncontrolled clinical trials of all time. Why? Let us count the ways by examining in greater depth the circumstances surrounding this particular doctor-patient relationship:

1. The patient was presenting with unusually severe symptoms; hence if nothing at all was done for her, the chances are that she would improve anyway in a few weeks due to the natural history of her pain cycle.

2. Dr. Smith, being an experienced physician, was (perhaps unconsciously) laying a strong foundation for a classic placebo effect to kick in here. Although he had appropriately included a disclaimer, he was suggesting to Mrs. Jones that acupuncture had an excellent chance to relieve her pain. Since she trusted her doctor, who had helped her many times before for many other illnesses, conditioning was operating to enhance her expectation of receiving pain relief. (If she were not amenable to the possibility that acupuncture would help her, she would also probably have politely declined Dr. Smith's kind offer to perform it on her in the first place.) Finally, since she was in a real state of distress, she had a strong desire for relief as well.

3. Because of the novelty of the treatment and Dr. Smith's request that she come in the next week so that he could monitor her progress and give her another treatment, Mrs. Jones unconsciously changed her behavior by returning home and being more compliant with Dr. Smith's other advice as well (e.g., taking her pain medication regularly, reducing the activities that she knew aggravated her condition, conscientiously wearing her

support hose, and spending more time with her legs elevated). In larger-scale clinical trials, this is sometimes called the Hawthorne effect, but more on this later.

4. To compound the situation, when she did return to Dr. Smith's office the following week, she was (as always) quite deferential to this authority figure to whom she felt greatly indebted for his kind service to her over the years. She was also naturally a very polite woman. Hence when Dr. Smith inquired if the acupuncture had helped, she would have been inclined to answer in the affirmative even if one of the above artifacts had not already kicked in to significantly reduce her pain. In the clinical trial business, this is sometimes called the good-subject syndrome (or, in behavioral research, a demand characteristic), but regardless of what it is called, it is something that, if not controlled in some way, is quite capable of inducing a clinician to make a false positive inference about his or her patient care.

So it was hardly surprising that when Dr. Smith asked her if the acupuncture was helping her, Mrs. Jones reported that her pain was much improved. And naturally our hero was quite pleased to hear this answer, being (as we know) a kind, conscientious man who genuinely wanted to help all of his patients, a motivation that had originally induced him to give up his vacation to study acupuncture. (Cognitive dissonance, which is nothing more than our absolute abhorrence to admitting our bad decisions, also could have operated here to keep Dr. Smith from suspecting that he might have traded a month in Aruba for a mediocre hotel room in Akron that smelled of cigarette smoke.) Anyway, because of this "incontrovertible" success (and it probably was initially a real success, even though its occurrence may have been due to things far removed from the small needles that had been inserted in Mrs. Jones's knee), Dr. Smith tried the procedure out on several other patients with similar success.

True, it didn't always work on everyone, and true, over time, even Mrs. Jones's pain seemed to return, but Dr. Smith's considerable clinical experience told him that no therapy was 100 percent effective 100 percent of the time. He nevertheless found his overall success rate to be encouraging. In other words, by the time the combination of Mrs. Jones's natural pain history, the Hawthorne effect, her natural politeness, and the placebo effect had begun to wear off, Dr. Smith had experienced enough additional clinical successes to allow him to rationalize a perfectly reasonable medical explanation for the gradually declining treatment effect for Mrs. Jones.

To illustrate why a physician who makes his living treating patients' symptoms might not know much about his successes and failures in this regard, let's return briefly to Sarah's story in chapter 3. At first glance these two "experimenters" would appear to have very little in common. After all, Sarah's failure to recognize the ineffectiveness of her therapy was facilitated by a placebo effect initiated by her trust in *Prevention* magazine's assurances that the therapy du jour might indeed prove effective, her belief that the answer was "out there," the natural history of her disease, and so forth. So far, then, Sarah's situation appears more relevant to Mrs. Jones's than to Dr. Smith's. Sarah's failure to remember all of the eventual failures of these therapies is, however, very similar to Dr. Smith's failure to question why the CAM therapy he was administering gradually lost its potency as well. And both failures are attributable to one simple fact: neither Sarah nor Dr. Smith collected data emanating from their little experiments, and hence neither could analyze what really happened.

I realize this conclusion may appear to border on the absurd, since no one, at least no one who isn't far past the point of no return on the obsessive-compulsive continuum, records the results of his or her day-to-day experiences. But by not recording the results accruing from their experiences, neither Sarah nor Dr. Smith ever came to the full realization that their therapies didn't really work in the first place (or have any long-term staying power).

In fact, from Sarah's perspective, most of her CAM therapies did work initially due to our now familiar list of inferential artifacts. And from Dr. Smith's perspective, acupuncture did help most of his patients. How did he know? Because they told him so, and why would they lie to their physician, of all people? And finally, even if these real, albeit artifactually induced, pain reduction effects did eventually wear off, both Sarah and Dr. Smith received some very real positive reinforcement for their experimental efforts in the form of initial successes, unnoticed or forgotten or rationalized failures, and hope—which in CAM really does spring eternal.

If, on the other hand, Sarah had charted her daily pain on something as simple as the visual analog scale depicted earlier, and if she had recorded the points in time at which she had tried each of her CAM therapies, she couldn't very well have avoided eventually catching a glimmer of what was actually going on.

The same holds for Dr. Smith, but very few physicians keep comparable data on the results of their clinical interventions. Thus Dr. Smith's continued belief in his CAM therapy of choice really is quite comparable to Sarah's continued acceptance of *Prevention*'s recommendations of CAM therapies and in some ways is more understandable. He, after all, was forced to rely upon his patients' truthfulness, plus he had many patients to monitor and he saw them only periodically. Even more problematic, physicians' judgments regarding their successes and failures have a serious built-in bias: patients who do not believe they are being helped tend not to come back. (This is very similar to an artifact called attrition that bedevils randomized clinical trials where research subjects who are not being helped tend to drop out of studies.)

So while acupuncture (like Sarah's therapies du jour) may have had no specific effect over and above the placebo effect and its accomplices, Dr. Smith (like Sarah) was continually reinforced for the attempt itself. And even if he did sometimes notice that eventually patients declined his offers of treatment or perhaps failed to show up for the next treatment, he saw lots of patients and very few of them were 100 percent compliant. And perhaps he even noticed that acupuncture eventually lost its effectiveness, but he had been in practice for many years and knew that nothing worked for a chronic condition 100 percent of the time. Perhaps, knowing this, he may have even occasionally suggested to patients that it was time to terminate this therapeutic approach and try something else, thereby employing rationalization to trump his cognitive dissonance.

Thus, like Sarah before him, the chances are that Dr. Smith was completely unaware of how such artifacts as natural history and/or his own psychological defense mechanisms operated to produce his false positive conclusion (or protect him from the truth). And he, even more than Sarah, would have almost certainly been insulted at the implication that his acupuncture treatments involved nothing more than a placebo effect. He had been trained to deliver his medical interventions in a positive, "in control" manner specifically designed to enhance the presumably effective (but often less than perfect) drugs he prescribed. He knew all about the placebo effect, and sometimes even knowingly imparted the expectation of success in patients to "trick" them into feeling better in those rare instances where no viable treatment options existed. In his mind, however, placebo effects were not the result of unconscious, unwitting actions on the part of physicians; they were actions that doctors carefully orchestrated, and their genesis was never, ever based upon physician ignorance.

Alas, placebo effects are ultimately built upon human frailty, and they depend upon ignorance (or misconceptions) for their continued effectiveness. Obviously a patient who knows that acupuncture has no specific effect is not going to be very receptive to allowing a physician to stick even very thin needles randomly into his or her body. Obviously, too, a physician who does not believe that acupuncture has any effect over and above the power of suggestion is not going to take the trouble to attend a time-consuming workshop in order to learn the complex intricacies involved in administering the therapy "correctly." It is the presence of these positive belief systems of both patients and their therapists, then, along with a few inferential impediments thrown in for good measure, that could explain the occurrence of those clinical benefits often attributed to CAM therapies. Their existence could also explain how and why such rituals have survived and tricked patients and therapists for millennia. In other words, the following conditions apply:

- Patient beliefs and expectations are necessary conditions for the placebo effect's occurrence, *and*

- These beliefs are, in turn, directly influenced by physician behaviors such as forcefulness and lack of equivocation, *and*

- These particular behaviors are further influenced by patient politeness as well as a real degree of benefit resulting from the placebo effect itself, *and*

- Both patients and physicians have a propensity to suffer from selective memory (we will see in Chapter 9 that research has shown that the placebo effect itself is associated with a certain genre of selective memory), *and*

- All of the above can be augmented by natural history, the Hawthorne effect, and attrition.

As a result, what we have is *an intricate feedback loop that, in the absence of systematically collected data, constitutes a continual impediment to clear reasoning.* In other words, what we really have here is a blueprint for a most wondrous, myth-perpetuating machine. And when an exclusively CAM-oriented patient seeks out a CAM therapist, the resulting dyadic relationship is undoubtedly an even more potent self-fulfilling prophecy, because in addition to all of the above, two more factors are involved:

- The CAM therapist's primary economic livelihood is at stake.

- The CAM therapist's self-concept, worldview, and professional identity depend upon the effectiveness of the therapy.

But just because people *can* be wrong about the effectiveness of something like CAM doesn't mean that they *are* wrong. What we are in dire need of at this point is some hard evidence on the topic, the production of which is the province of science, which over the years has developed a specialized set of statistical and procedural strategies that allow us to collect and analyze data to facilitate our very human need for making correct inferences and drawing causal conclusions under even the most difficult of conditions.

And since a considerable amount of scientific research now exists regarding the effectiveness of CAM therapies, it would seem that it should be a simple matter to review this evidence and arrive at a definitive conclusion. Yet these results cannot be interpreted without a basic understanding of how research in general is conducted and, more important, how it can go awry.

CHAPTER FIVE

Impediments That Prevent Poorly Trained Scientists from Making Valid Inferences

Even if ordinary people (such as Sarah) and the physicians who treat them (such as Dr. Smith) have major impediments to overcome in order to figure out what does and doesn't work, it's ultimately not up to them to evaluate issues scientifically. Ordinary people and clinicians didn't come up with the theory of evolution or discover that a specific type of bread mold can cure syphilis. That sort of work—to determine the cause of things as well as what is good for us—is what we have scientists for, isn't it?

It is, but if they are not very, very careful, even our best-trained scientists are capable of being tricked by exactly the same phenomena that confounded Sarah's and Dr. Smith's little experiments. And unfortunately, in a discipline such as CAM, which is well outside mainstream scientific inquiry, most of its researchers historically have not been that well trained. Allow me to illustrate some of the implications of this circumstance via the further adventures of Dr. Smith.

THE RETURN OF DR. SMITH

As a graphic illustration of how bad things sometimes happen to good people, our old friend Dr. Smith suffered a professionally traumatic experience soon after his appearance in the last chapter. When invited to a professional conference to present a paper on some of his clinical experiences in treating patients with acupuncture, he was questioned by an unusually boorish biostatistician (so unlike your civil, easygoing author) who leveled a number of criticisms at his conclusions. Most of these criticisms took the form of complaining about Dr. Smith's reliance upon only his clinical experiences with selected patients in the absence of any real data.

Not being one to take such attacks on his clinical judgment lightly, Dr. Smith decided to conduct his own research study in collaboration with a colleague from a nearby medical school. This individual helped Dr. Smith design his experiment and shepherded it through his university's institutional review board himself.[1]

Given Dr. Smith's professional interests, Dr. Smith and in keeping with the previously conducted acupuncture research with which the two were familiar, the patient symptom that they chose to employ as their outcome measure was pain (measured using the same visual analog scale depicted earlier). The medical condition was osteoarthritis of the knee, and the therapy was, of course, acupuncture.

In designing their trial, Dr. Smith and his colleague ran across several options used in the design of studies by past acupuncture researchers, but, being pragmatists, they decided that the most natural and straightforward way to conduct their experiment was as follows (and as summarized in Figure 5.1):

- Mention the availability of the experiment to Dr. Smith's patients and post a sign about it near the elevator in the university hospital's parking garage as a way of soliciting other patients to participate in the study

- Screen interested patients over the phone to ensure that they qualified for the study (which meant they had to have osteoarthritis in at least one knee and had to be experiencing a considerable degree of pain—defined as 3 or more on a visual analog scale ranging from 1 to 10)

- Invite qualifying patients to come to Dr. Smith's office in order to sign an informed consent statement, fill out some questionnaires, and be examined to ensure that they did indeed have osteoarthritis of the knee

- Schedule the qualifying participants' acupuncture sessions

- Administer the actual acupuncture treatment

- Obtain follow-up pain information on the participants once the requisite acupuncture sessions had been completed

- Once the trial is completed, get someone to analyze the data, write up the results, and make travel arrangements for the next year's Nobel Prize ceremony in Stockholm

Dr. Smith reasoned that if the patients' pain decreased following their acupuncture treatment (that is, at the follow-up pain assessment compared to the baseline assessment) and if they did not change their medication or receive any new treatments during this time period, then at the very least he would be able to serve an ample helping of crow to his critics at his association's next annual meeting. He would, after all, now have hard data from a reasonably large number of patients collected under standardized conditions to replace his previous clinical experiences. If his study was properly conducted, it would surely prove what he already knew to be the case—that acupuncture would result in decreased pain for his participants (because he had personally observed this with his own patients), which in turn would mean that no one could now find any fault with his inference that acupuncture was indeed effective (if not the long-sought panacea) for reducing arthritis pain.

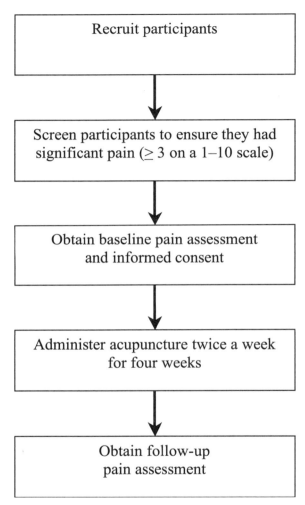

Figure 5.1. Dr. Smith's Acupuncture Trial

Table 5.1. Results of Dr. Smith's Acupuncture Trial

Participant	First Pain Assessment	Second Pain Assessment	Pain Reduction
Patient 1	5.4	4.4	−1.0
Patient 2	4.9	4.2	−0.7
Patient 3	5.6	3.7	−1.9
Patient 4	5.5	3.7	−1.8
Patient 5	8.6	5.1	−3.5
Patient 6	9.0	5.3	−3.7
Patient 7	10.0	5.8	−4.2
Patient 8	10.0	5.8	−4.2
Average	7.4	4.8	−2.6

And to top the whole thing off, he was absolutely correct! In fact, the actual results obtained are presented in Table 5.1 (although, naturally, a real trial would have a few more participants than this).

Dr. Smith even obtained the services of a biostatistician, who wrote the following sentence for him to insert in his paper: "As determined by a dependent samples *t*-test ($t = 5.2$ [7], $p = .001$), the participants' pain significantly declined following four weeks of acupuncture treatment." Dr. Smith was ecstatic at this statistical blessing, so he formally applied to present the results of his study to his professional organization the next year, and his paper was accepted. Needless to say, he and his colleague felt very good about their results and prepared for the redemptive approbation of their peers this time around.

Ah, the perversity of life! The truth of the matter is that despite all his efforts, his critics were destined to be even more caustic this time. Why? Because he was now invoking the authority of science in support of his earlier conclusions based upon the results of a severely flawed experiment. Since no one enjoys the actual details of a good person's suffering, I won't reveal what transpired at Dr. Smith's presentation. Instead, let's simply examine the inferential flaws that would almost surely conspire to ensure that his experiment produced false positive conclusions.

THE NATURAL HISTORY OF CHRONIC PAIN

We've already discussed natural history as it related to Sarah Cohen's experiences and to Dr. Smith's clinical practice. Sarah, it will be remembered, was much more likely to try out one of *Prevention* magazine's CAM interventions when her pain was bothering her the most. By the same token, Dr. Smith's patients were much more likely to come to see him when they were in the most pain, and as a compassionate man, he was more likely to offer acupuncture to them at that point.

So why wouldn't the same phenomenon operate for people who volunteered to participate in a clinical trial? Wouldn't most people be more likely to commit the necessary time and effort involved in participating in an experiment when their pain was near the apex of their natural history cycle? Just in case there was an exception or two to this rule, Dr. Smith and his colleague effectively plugged this loophole by only permitting individuals to volunteer who were experiencing a significant amount of knee pain from osteoarthritis (which, it will be remembered, involved not permitting anyone with pain less than a 3 on a 1–10 visual analog scale to participate).

Thus if we assume that the depiction of the natural history of Sarah's osteoarthritis pain was a relatively common one and constituted an accurate characterization of osteoarthritis patients in general, why wouldn't the same artifact occur for a group of Sarahs? Especially since, as is standard practice in research involving pain, patients were allowed into a trial only if they were experiencing a significant amount of pain?[2]

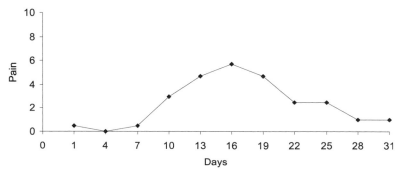

Figure 5.2. Revisiting the Natural History of Sarah's Arthritis Pain

Well, the answer is that the artifact *can* occur for a group of people just as easily as it can occur for a single individual. For illustrative purposes only, let's assume an admittedly strange scenario in which a group of patients with a natural history of pain almost identical to Sarah's showed up to volunteer for Dr. Smith's trial, which, you will remember, took the form redepicted here in Figure 5.2.

Now of course everyone wouldn't show up in Dr. Smith's office at the same point in this cycle. If the potential participants arrived independently of how much pain they were feeling, then everyone at days 1–9 and days 22–31 would be thanked for their interest and sent home because they didn't qualify. Individuals at the equivalent of days 10–21, however, would be accepted with open arms.

In real life many of these people would naturally wait until their pain was either near its zenith or ascending toward it, but the end result would be the same. Even if Dr. Smith never even got around to administering his cherished acupuncture intervention (for reasons that will soon be apparent), he might very well have achieved results something like those shown in Figure 5.3.

And his biostatistician would probably still bless these results with statistical significance, since he would never suspect that no one received any treatment at all.

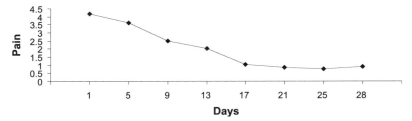

Figure 5.3. Hypothetical Results Due to Natural History for Patients Allowed to Enter the Study Only Between Days 10 and 21 of the Pain Cycle
The entire pain cycle is shown in Figure 5.2

REGRESSION TO THE MEAN

While the actual profile I've painted here of the natural history of Sarah's pain may be a bit stylized (few natural phenomena occur with such regularity and predictability), there is an experimental artifact that inevitably occurs when an experiment begins at a time in which participant symptoms are either unusually high or unusually low. Known as regression to the mean, it looks and operates very much like the hypothetically truncated natural history pattern depicted in Figure 5.3, but occurs whether the symptom involved is cyclical in nature or a one-time phenomenon. Recognized by researchers for at least 120 years, regression to the mean is a purely statistical phenomenon that results from two factors: the group being looked at ranks unusually high or low on the outcome of interest (in this case, patients who volunteered because they are experiencing pain at a level that is extreme compared to the larger population to which they belong), and the variables involved are not perfectly correlated (perfect correlation never occurs in reality anyway, but in this case the imperfectness is due to a large extent to the imprecision in the way the outcome of interest, pain, is measured).[3] The phenomenon is rather counterintuitive, but what's most relevant here is that, unlike many of the other artifacts we've discussed, regression to the mean is not something that *may* occur to confound a study. It is something that *will* always occur with mathematical predictability as long as the two conditions just discussed occur.

INVESTIGATOR DISINGENUOUSNESS

There is an entire class of experimental artifacts that is quite easily understood by anyone with no research training at all other than experience in life itself. However, their occurrence, by definition, is something that only the people integrally related to a trial ever know about.

We know full well that Dr. Smith would never knowingly misrepresent anything, but a lot of strange things can happen at the point at which investigators start to write up the results of their trials. It is not unusual for a trial, for example, to include multiple (sometimes a dozen or more) outcome variables. Good research practice requires that at the beginning of the trial an investigator specify one of these variables as the primary endpoint, which means that it is the main outcome variable that will be used to determine whether or not the study produced positive or negative results.

The problem is that in most cases no one other than the investigator was around when this outcome was selected, and even if a record exists in the original grant proposal, no one ever bothers to go back and look. Think what a temptation it is, then, after spending a few years of one's life supervising the conduct of a trial, to change the designation of an a priori specified primary outcome if no effect is found for it but one is found for a related outcome. Who is to know? And is it really that important anyway?

Or suppose that the outcome measures were assessed at several time points but statistical significance was found at only a few of these. It is very easy for investigators to convince themselves in hindsight that all of these time points weren't really necessary or even appropriate. So why even mention the ones at which a significant effect wasn't obtained?

Or what about glitches in carrying out the experimental protocol? These could include accidentally revealing to participants or to clinicians administering the treatments who in the study was receiving the active treatment and who was receiving the placebo treatment. Is it really necessary to mention things such as this in the actual journal article? Or if a large number of participants drop out of the study before it is completed, why not simply exclude mention of attrition and hope that the journal editor and reviewers don't notice (especially since doing so may preclude acceptance of the manuscript in a high-impact research journal)?

The list goes on and on, but the bottom line is the same. The vast majority of these practices conspire to produce false positive results, and in the final analysis, the main protection we have against these practices is our reliance upon the investigator's integrity and commitment to scientific transparency.[4]

THE HAWTHORNE EFFECT: KNOWING BIG BROTHER IS WATCHING

We all behave differently when we know that we are being watched, and participating in a clinical trial involves some very intensive "watching." One well-publicized example of this a few years ago involved researchers observing hand-washing behavior in public bathrooms. Victims who didn't know they were being observed were considerably less likely to wash their hands after using the toilet than those who knew they weren't alone in the bathroom.[5]

An even more famous instance of this phenomenon (at least from the perspective of the history of science) occurred in an industrial experiment in which the very act of observing (and measuring) workers' productivity caused them to work harder to increase their output. Dubbed the Hawthorne effect after the Western Electric Company plant in which the study occurred, this phenomenon soon came to represent a tendency for experimental participants to behave differently when they know they are in a trial.[6]

And if that weren't enough, trial participants not only behave differently but have a tendency to provide experimenters with what they think the experimenters want to hear. They also tend to behave in more socially acceptable ways, such as in the hand-washing experiment, and sometimes even to behave more sensibly, such as by taking their pre-scribed medications more conscientiously or avoiding activities that they know exacerbate their conditions. Moreover, the very act of volunteer-ing for a trial may produce a level of cognitive dissonance among par-ticipants sufficient for them to convince themselves that they improved as a function of the experience (and all the inconvenience it entailed). While these genres of artifacts are known by a wide variety of names, they almost always operate to produce positive results that have nothing to do with the interventions or therapies being evaluated; they operate completely independently from (and in addition to) natural history; and they are especially likely to occur in experiments where the experimental outcomes are subjective self-reports (of which, alas, pain is a quintessential example).[7]

EXPERIMENTER BIAS

But there is another, even more serious problem with Dr. Smith's little study, and that is Dr. Smith himself. Because Dr. Smith obviously knew that everyone in his trial was receiving acupuncture, and since he des-perately wanted his trial to produce positive results (if for no other reason that the fact that he was a compassionate man who genuinely wanted to help his patients), it would have been very difficult for him to interact with his study participants in a completely dispassionate manner. It would also have been very difficult for him to avoid biasing his exper-iment unconsciously by letting his patients feel how important their welfare was to him and how much he hoped that what he was doing in this trial would contribute positively to their well-being. Perhaps he might even have unconsciously prescribed a higher-than-usual dose of arthritis medication for one of his patients whom he knew was experi-encing pain during the course of the study. Perhaps his longtime office secretary, who knew how important the trial was to her old friend (and employer), might even have thrown in some not-so-subtle hints to that effect when she collected the participants' final pain data.

The primary way we have to prevent these unconscious, uncontrolled sources of bias is via experimental blinding, where neither the individuals who collect data nor the individuals who provide the experimental treatment know which patients are receiving the treatment. Of course, there is no way to avoid bias of this type in a single-group experiment.

Still, experimenter bias of this genre, which is independent of (and additive to) natural history, regression to the mean, and the Hawthorne effect, pales into insignificance in the presence of the mother of all experimental artifacts, the placebo effect.

THE PLACEBO EFFECT

In the last two chapters we saw how the placebo effect can conspire to cloud both patients' and practitioners' judgments. It is equally pernicious in clinical research and can make complete fools out of scientists. In an area such as CAM, it is the most successful of all inferential threats in producing false positive results. It is also absolutely impossible to control in a single-group study such as Dr. Smith's acupuncture trial. In fact, it cannot be controlled in any CAM trial that does not employ a control group of some sort that is capable of tricking its members into thinking they are getting a CAM therapy. Thus, for an acupuncture trial, a credible fake acupuncture procedure must be devised that people can't distinguish from real acupuncture. In a chiropractic trial, a fake spinal manipulation of some sort must be devised and tested until it is demonstrated to be indistinguishable from the real thing.

Why? Because participants generally will not volunteer to participate in a CAM trial in the first place if they do not believe that the CAM therapy in question has a chance to help them. Thus in Dr. Smith's trial, most of the participating patients would indeed have experienced less pain as a function of these beliefs each time they received acupuncture. They would, in other words, have experienced a placebo effect as a function of their expectations, regardless of whether or not the presence of little needles in various parts of their body had any specific effect on pain.

What makes matters even worse is that the placebo effect is tacked onto the effects of everything else we've discussed that conspires to produce false positive results. Therefore, a trained scientist reading a report of a CAM trial designed like Dr. Smith's that did *not* report positive results would be shocked and would suspect that one of six things was operating:

1. The therapy was actually harmful.
2. The disease being investigated was so degenerative that afflicted patients got worse from the disease itself.
3. So few participants were employed that statistical significance was not possible.
4. The trial was conducted so badly that its results were completely invalid.
5. The results were fraudulent.
6. The investigator's negative attitude toward acupuncture biased the results, which is highly unlikely since no one can conduct an acupuncture trial without an acupuncturist and acupuncturists by definition have a positive attitude toward their therapies.

So in retrospect, it is probably obvious that Dr. Smith *should* have designed his little trial in such a way that the placebo effect and its nefarious siblings couldn't completely ruin all of his hard work and subject him to the professional abuse of boorish biostatisticians. But take heart. Since Dr. Smith is a fictional character, there is no reason why we can't afford him one final chance at redemption. And in so doing, we can explore how the effectiveness of a CAM therapy *should* be evaluated— which of course is to employ a randomized, controlled trial employing a credible placebo control group.

CHAPTER SIX

Why Randomized Placebo Control Groups Are Necessary in CAM Research

Employing a placebo control group does not prevent the placebo effect from occurring. The only way to do that is to convince people that the experimental intervention that they are about to receive will *not* help them or that there is nothing special about it. Using a placebo group doesn't even tell us how large the placebo effect is in a particular experiment because so many other inferential impediments are operating at the same time. The only way to ascertain the actual size of a placebo effect is to employ a no-treatment control group and to compare its results with those obtained for the placebo group.

In short, what the use of a placebo control accomplishes is to permit the experimenter to ascertain the size of the placebo effect *plus* its extended family of artifacts is (such as natural history and the Hawthorne effect) and then to "subtract" these extraneous effects from those obtained for the experimental intervention. This is possible only if the experimental participants, the clinicians who deliver the treatments (including the placebo), *and* the research staff can be prevented from knowing which participants are receiving the real therapy and which participants are receiving the placebo. Unfortunately, in most CAM trials other than homeopathy, it is extremely difficult to construct placebos that prevent participants from guessing their group assignment, and it is patently impossible to blind most types of therapists. The result is that the placebo effect is either uncontrolled or only partially controlled, thereby seriously undermining the validity of the trials' results.

To the extent that these difficulties can be surmounted, randomized, placebo-controlled trials are far and away our best line of defense against the production of false positive results—the bane of all trials, but especially in areas such as CAM, where the placebo effect is such a persistent impediment to arriving at a correct inference regarding which therapies are and are not effective. Unless the trial is very, very competently run, however, the inclusion of a randomized, placebo-controlled group isn't a foolproof strategy because there are some sources of bias upon which the randomization of patients to real and placebo therapies has little or no effect. But basically this is all we have, so let's illustrate some of a placebo's strengths and weaknesses via Dr. Smith's second trial.

DR. SMITH'S REVENGE

Something that I might have forgotten to mention about Dr. Smith is that since childhood he had been afflicted with a relatively severe (but, until recently, manageable) case of obsessive-compulsive disorder. So following his second bashing at the annual meeting of his professional society, he girded his loins and went back to the drawing board in order to conduct a randomized, placebo-controlled acupuncture trial.

Before we go into all of that, let's review the results, repeated here in Table 6.1, that he obtained from his earlier, star-crossed trial in which he employed no control group at all.

Of course it's a mere coincidence that he obtained an improvement in this initial trial of 35 percent ($2.6 \div 7.4$), exactly as Henry Beecher would have predicted. But otherwise these are fake numbers, since even Dr. Smith wouldn't conduct a trial with only eight patients, nor (I hope)

Table 6.1. Results of Dr. Smith's First Acupuncture Trial

Participant	First Pain Assessment	Second Pain Assessment	Pain Reduction
Patient 1	5.4	4.4	−1.0
Patient 2	4.9	4.2	−0.7
Patient 3	5.6	3.7	−1.9
Patient 4	5.5	3.7	−1.8
Patient 5	8.6	5.1	−3.5
Patient 6	9.0	5.3	−3.7
Patient 7	10.0	5.8	−4.2
Patient 8	10.0	5.8	−4.2
Average	7.4	4.8	−2.6

would any arthritis patients anywhere report pain as high as 10.0 on a 1–10 scale.

Nevertheless, learning from his previous mistakes, our hero proceeded to redesign his trial. This time around he went to a CAM research center and learned how to administer a sham acupuncture procedure that had been demonstrated to be fairly difficult for participants to distinguish from the real thing (there aren't any that are perfect). He also recruited patients as he did before, but took the added precaution of randomly assigning these patients to two groups: one that received the sham procedure and one that received the same acupuncture treatment that was administered in the first study.[1]

Let's see what Dr. Smith's results might look like if acupuncture really is a placebo therapy—that is, if it has no effect at all upon pain over and above the placebo effect and its partners in crime. Let's further assume that he wound up with exactly the same pain results as he achieved in the first trial, except this time four of his patients were randomly chosen to receive real acupuncture and four were randomly chosen to receive fake (or placebo) acupuncture.[2] The results of the second trial appear in Table 6.2.

In this case, we have an entirely different inferential scenario in which four of the original patients (numbers 2, 3, 6, and 7) received nothing but our experimental artifacts (natural history, the placebo effect, and the Hawthorne effect), while the remaining four (numbers 1, 4, 5, and 8) also received these artifacts plus the experimental intervention (real acupuncture). Everyone still improved, just as they did in the uncontrolled trial, but now the presence of a randomized, placebo-controlled group will force Dr. Smith to interpret his results in a radically different

Table 6.2. An Illustration of How a Randomized, Placebo-Controlled Group Controls for Natural History, the Hawthorne Effect, and Placebo Effects

Participant	Baseline	Follow-up	Pain Reduction
Acupuncture Group			
Patient 1	5.4	4.4	−1.0
Patient 4	5.5	3.7	−1.8
Patient 5	8.6	5.1	−3.5
Patient 8	10.0	5.8	−4.2
Acupuncture average	7.4	4.8	−2.6
Placebo Group			
Patient 2	4.9	4.2	−0.7
Patient 3	5.6	3.7	−1.9
Patient 6	9.0	5.3	−3.7
Patient 7	10.0	5.8	−4.2
Placebo average	7.4	4.8	−2.6

way. (Or it will force his biostatistician to force him to interpret them differently.)

Why? Because everybody's pain still improved as a function of our nemeses. Patients 2, 3, 6, and 7 theoretically did not know that they were in the placebo group; hence they should be the beneficiaries of the same placebo effect as Patients 1, 4, 5, and 8. Now, however, the question of interest is no longer whether people who received acupuncture improved. Instead, the relevant question becomes:

Did people who received acupuncture improve more than people who received the placebo?

The answer should be obvious: no. The study's interpretation should be equally obvious:

For patients suffering from osteoarthritis of the knee, acupuncture does not result in a greater reduction of pain than a placebo.

Why? Because the difference between the average changes in pain experienced by the acupuncture group minus the average changes in pain experienced by the placebo group $(2.6 - 2.6 = 0)$ equals the pain relief due to acupuncture. Why? Because if the trial were competently run, both groups received equal shots of placebo, natural history, regression to the mean, and Hawthorne effects.

This, then, is the true beauty of the logic behind the use of a randomized, placebo-controlled trial. But just because an investigator understands this logic doesn't mean that he or she can emotionally accept it when it violates his or her personal worldview. Complementary and alternative medicine, like the placebo effect, is really more about belief than logic. And that, dear reader, underscores something that a placebo can't control: the emotions and beliefs of not only those who practice CAM but sometimes also those who investigate its effectiveness.

What else other than "Acupuncture is no more effective than a placebo for reducing the pain or osteoarthritis of the knee" could Dr. Smith have concluded, after all? But would it really come as a shock that he still believed that acupuncture was effective, even after conducting his very own placebo-controlled trial?

It shouldn't surprise us at all, at least if we put ourselves in Dr. Smith's shoes. He is a fervent believer in acupuncture. He has a very real and very strong commitment to helping people. He has gone to a great deal of trouble to conduct this trial, perhaps soliciting funding for it by submitting a grant proposal and personally lobbying (or calling in some favors from his fellow medical school alumni to lobby) the funding agency to accept his proposal. He had even announced to all of his skeptical colleagues (including his boorish conference critic) that he was mounting a randomized, controlled trial to verify his clinical experiences.

Now, therefore, not only does he feel that his professional credibility is on the line, but his faith in acupuncture has actually grown as a result of conducting this trial. Previously he has witnessed acupuncture work with his own eyes in his private practice, but now he has demonstrated that it works in a randomized, placebo-controlled trial in which all of his acupuncture patients improved at least one entire scale point. So what if patients 2, 3, 6, and 7 also improved? There are plenty of ways to explain this, according to Dr. Smith's reasoning, and the truth of the matter is that he never completely understood nor trusted the esoteric, stylistic dance steps involved in conducting a randomized, controlled trial anyway. After all, perhaps the placebo acupuncture procedure was somehow therapeutic in and of itself. What else could explain the fact that all the patients who received it improved?

There are ample precedents for such an interpretation. Consider an actual example from the medical literature published in the refereed journal *Complementary Therapies in Medicine*. The investigators of this study (faculty members from a German medical school) duly reported that they had conducted a "prospective, randomized, controlled, patient- and investigator-blinded clinical trial" involving a two-group design very similar to our hypothetical study: "Group 1 (treatment) had traditional needle placement and manipulation, whereas in group 2 (control) needles were placed away from classic positions and not manipulated."

The investigators found very similar results to those in Table 6.2, although they employed more participants (sixty-seven in all) and they were investigating pain due to osteoarthritis of the hip rather than of the knee. Instead of having the temerity to suggest that acupuncture might not be the long-sought panacea for arthritis pain, however, they concluded that acupuncture was indeed effective:

> We conclude from these results that needle placement in the area of the affected hip is associated with improvement in the symptoms of osteoarthritis. It appears to be less important to follow the rules of traditional acupuncture techniques.[3]

Had these investigators never heard of natural history, regression to the mean, or the Hawthorne effect? If not, they certainly should not be conducting clinical trials, because they simply don't have the training necessary to conduct them well or to interpret the results in a way that factors in critical variables. But if they are familiar with such things as natural history, then they still should not be conducting clinical trials, because their conclusions are disingenuous at best. At the very least we know that they had heard of the placebo effect, because they employed a fake acupuncture group to control for it. (And they did so successfully, which is why there was no difference between the real and fake acupuncture groups.) Unfortunately, as will be illustrated in Chapter 11, even some of our top journals have begun to allow CAM researchers to pretend that their placebo control groups are really treatment groups involving nonspecific effects (which you will remember is how the placebo effect is normally defined), hence neatly explaining why they obtain no difference between their CAM therapy and placebo control. Naturally interpretative bias of this nature unnecessarily complicates the provision of a straightforward answer to the very straightforward question we are ultimately interested in answering:

> *Is any CAM therapy more effective than a placebo?*

I think any adequately trained, experienced investigator would characterize practices such as this as disingenuous. It is comparable to a pharmaceutical company, upon finding no difference between the drug they hope to market and the placebo they have used to evaluate it, making the argument that both of their treatments, their new drug and the placebo, helped people. Can anyone anywhere imagine the Food and Drug Administration then giving the pharmaceutical company permission to market both their drug and placebo based upon such evidence? If it did, I wonder how much the drug company would charge for the placebo.

PROBLEMS THAT EVEN RANDOMLY ASSIGNED PLACEBO GROUPS CAN'T PREVENT

Biased (or incompetent) researchers aren't the only problem one encounters when attempting to interpret the evidence produced by CAM research (and to be fair, conventional medical research as well). Even when conducted by an experienced investigator, it is not uncommon for a randomized, placebo-controlled trial to produce false positive results. (I sometimes think that it was anticipation of the very real difficulties inherent in running a competent randomized, placebo-controlled trial that originally inspired both the old English proverb "There's many a slip twixt the cup and the lip" and Murphy's even more eloquent pronouncement: "Anything that can go wrong will go wrong.")

Far and away the most difficult aspect of such an endeavor involves ensuring the credibility of the placebo. It is a lot easier to report in a research journal that patients, clinicians, and data collectors were blinded with respect to group assignment than it is to actually prevent these patients, clinicians, data collectors, and statisticians from really knowing who is receiving which treatment—especially patients.[4] There are a number of reasons for this difficulty, but two of the biggest culprits involve incidental cues such as side effects and the informed consent process.

Side Effects

While it is difficult enough to blind patients in any type of trial, it is much more difficult to keep participants in the dark in a trial involving procedures (such as acupuncture, chiropractic manipulation, or surgery) than in, say, a drug trial.[5] Even so, it is not all that simple even in drug trials involving placebo capsules identical in appearance, smell, and taste to the real drug. Patients are often able to tell what they are getting solely by the side effects that most drugs produce. It is true that patients in placebo groups experience side effects themselves (one estimate is between 4 and 26 percent of patients), but heavy-duty pharmaceuticals often produce heavy-duty side effects that can make group assignment pretty obvious to their recipients.[6]

While side effects of this nature shouldn't be that problematic for any CAM therapies that really are ineffective (and thus nothing more than placebos themselves), they often involve even more obvious cues emanating from the fact that something actually being done to one's body is difficult not to notice. Acupuncture, after all, *feels* like someone is sticking sharp little needles into one's body, so if someone only pretends to do so, the patient is quite likely to figure this out by the end of the trial. Needles can be inserted in irrelevant parts of the body in the placebo group, as was done in the German study above, but then the critics—or the investigators themselves—can claim that these irrelevant needles were somehow therapeutic. Furthermore, even Robert De Niro might have a difficult time not unconsciously communicating to his patients which treatment they were receiving, real or fake. (Acupuncturists, after all, aren't accustomed to knowingly administering a bogus therapy.) And other CAM procedures, such as the spinal realignment practiced by chiropractors, can be even more problematic.

What, then, is the ultimate effect of all this? That only some of the participants are fooled some of the time, hence the placebo group experiences only a partial placebo effect and the experimental group receives a full dose thereof. Which means, in turn, that all single-blinded CAM studies (i.e., studies in which the therapists know to which group the participants have been assigned) begin with a positive bias toward the real treatment regardless of whether the investigators themselves are biased or not.

Informed Consent

While not often conceptualized as an impediment to interpreting the results of randomized, controlled trials, it would certainly be a lot easier to conduct CAM research if it weren't necessary to tell participants so much about the trials they are volunteering for. Decades of abuse, however, such as enrolling educationally disadvantaged African Americans in lifelong syphilis studies and not even telling them they had the disease[7] or coercing parents of institutionalized mentally retarded children to allow fecal extracts to be injected in their bodies to induce hepatitis by telling them that they would have to take care of their children themselves if they didn't agree to allow their children to be experimented upon has made it absolutely imperative that people know exactly what they are volunteering for.[8]

So today an investigator such as Dr. Smith is required—and rightly so, by the way—to have his experimental participants sign a statement that contains some variant of the following clause:

> You will be assigned by the computer to either receive eight 30-minute acupuncture treatments (two per week for four weeks) or the same number of "fake" acupuncture treatments in which the needles will not actually be inserted in your body.

While there are considerable differences from institution to institution regarding how much of the experimental protocol must be disclosed to participants, the statement would then go on to describe potential side effects of acupuncture along with other aspects of the trial. And again, while acupuncture doesn't normally have many side effects other than minor pain associated with the procedure and the occasional accident in which the needles are inserted too deeply, the possibility of these adverse incidents would have to be explained prior to the participants' entry into the study, which means that *the informed consent process itself has at least one significant side effect:* it heightens participants' awareness that not only may they not receive the treatment for which they signed up, but they may receive something utterly worthless. What this means is that a trial such as Dr. Smith's has a built-in incentive for participants to try to figure out which treatment they are receiving. After all, it is a lot to ask someone to perhaps drive an hour or so eight times during the next month to receive an intentionally worthless treatment.

As an example, let's revisit Dr. Smith's seemingly well-designed study as a way of illustrating what the implications are of patients gradually becoming aware of their group assignments over the course of a trial. Returning to the data in Table 6.2, the participants in both groups will still improve over time because of natural history, regression to the mean, and the Hawthorne effect, if nothing else. Now, however, let's assume that patient blinding was compromised somewhat over the course of the trial. To the extent that this happens (and in my experience it usually does in placebo-controlled CAM trials), the placebo effect will operate more strongly for the real acupuncture group than for the placebo group regardless of whether the real treatment is effective or not.

To illustrate, let's consider our four real acupuncture recipients. They will most likely improve a little more by the end of the trial because now they are much more convinced that they are receiving real acupuncture than was the case at the beginning of the study. How would this happen? Perhaps because they felt those sharp little pinpricks, or because the acupuncturist was so enthusiastic, or because the acupuncturist performed the procedure so confidently.

And of course the opposite would be true of our poor placebo patients. They will now have some serious doubts regarding whether or not they are really getting true acupuncture. Perhaps they began to notice that the sharp little pinpricks mentioned in their informed consent statement never materialized, or the acupuncturist seemed to be a little embarrassed when pretending to insert the needles, or the therapist was somewhat inept at this bogus procedure or communicated misgivings through some subtle difference in body language or verbal cues (which wouldn't occur in a well-designed drug trial because the people handing out the capsules really don't know which intervention they are administering).

Whatever the case, let's assume, due to incomplete blinding, that the placebo patients only got 50 percent of their original pain relief. The results appear in Table 6.3.

Table 6.3. The Results of Imperfect Blinding: Why Even Randomized Trials Can't Prevent False Positive Results if Participants Can Guess Their Group Assignments

Participant	Baseline	Partial Blinding Add-on Effect*	Follow-up	Pain Reduction
Acupuncture Group				
Patient 1	5.4	NA	4.4	−1.0
Patient 4	5.5	NA	3.7	−1.8
Patient 5	8.6	NA	5.1	−3.5
Patient 8	10.0	NA	5.8	−4.2
Acupuncture average	7.4	NA	4.8	−2.6
Placebo Group				
Patient 2	4.9	+0.35	4.55	−0.35
Patient 3	5.6	+0.95	4.65	−0.95
Patient 6	9.0	+1.85	7.15	−1.85
Patient 7	10.0	+2.1	7.9	−2.1
Placebo average	7.4	+1.3	6.1	−1.3

Computed by assuming that the control group's pain relief would decrease by 50 percent (because most of the participants now realized that they were not receiving the experimental intervention and hence do not receive the full benefit of a placebo effect). Results rounded to nearest five-hundredth.

While the effect is not nearly as dramatic as was the case for Dr. Smith's original single-group study, there is now a pain reduction difference favoring the acupuncture group despite the experimenters' best efforts at controlling for the placebo effect. If a biostatistician blessed these results as being statistically significant, even the most rigorous journals would embrace the conclusion that *acupuncture is more effective than a placebo for reducing the pain due to osteoarthritis of the knee*. And if these relatively unimpressive results were found in a trial containing only eight participants per group, the computer *would* indeed indicate that these tiny differences between the two groups were statistically significant. This, in turn, would allow Dr. Smith to continue administering acupuncture to his patients and perhaps even become a force in the growth industry known as CAM.

Experimental Attrition

There is, however, an even more problematic consequence of this growing awareness of group membership over the course of a trial: experimental attrition. This very common artifact is one of the most serious inferential pitfalls that can befall a randomized trial—especially if the dropout rate exceeds 20–25 percent.

It would take a very strange group of people who suffered daily pain and who volunteered their time and effort to participate in a trial to actually prefer to be assigned to a placebo control group. Many, in fact, begin to drop out of the trial once they suspect that they *are* receiving a placebo—especially if they are either feeling worse or failing to witness any improvement. While it is a rare trial in which none of the participants drops out, studies in which large proportions do so are especially problematic to interpret. To illustrate, let's examine what would happen if only one participant in Dr. Smith's study dropped out. The most likely candidate would be patient 7, since we already know that the blinding for this trial is less than perfect (hence participants in the placebo group are more likely to drop out than their counterparts in the acupuncture group) and that this individual was suffering more pain from the outset than anyone else in the placebo group. The effects of patient 7's departure on the trial are shown in Table 6.4.

Now we have a much more pronounced difference between the acupuncture and placebo groups with attrition than we had without it. Even if we hadn't had the artificial luxury of knowing that this patient would have improved more than anyone else in the placebo group, we might have *suspected* this outcome given our knowledge of natural

Table 6.4. An Illustration of What Happens When Trial Participants Guess They Are in the Placebo Group and Leave the Study

Participant	Baseline	Partial Blinding Add-on Effect	Follow-up	Pain Reduction
Acupuncture Group				
Patient 1	5.4	NA	4.4	−1.0
Patient 4	5.5	NA	3.7	−1.8
Patient 5	8.6	NA	5.1	−3.5
Patient 8	10.0	NA	5.8	−4.2
Acupuncture average	7.4	NA	4.8	−2.6
Placebo Group				
Patient 2	4.9	+0.35	4.55	−0.35
Patient 3	5.6	+0.95	4.65	−0.95
Patient 6	9.0	+1.85	7.15	−1.85
Patient 7	NA	NA	NA	NA
Placebo average with attrition	6.5	+1.05	5.45	−1.05
Placebo average without attrition	7.4	+1.3	6.1	−1.3

history. But in science our expectations don't count for much, so if these results had occurred in an actual trial, we would have been forced to conclude that acupuncture resulted in even greater pain reduction compared to a placebo effect than the results depicted in Table 6.3. And even if the trial's investigator had dutifully noted the interpretive limitations inherent in the degree of attrition observed, neither the headlines in the newspaper nor the news report of the study likely would have mentioned the problem.

So randomized, placebo-controlled trials can be worse than useless unless they are conducted very, very carefully under the best of circumstances. And evaluating a CAM therapy that involves a procedure, as opposed to a pill, is far from the best of circumstances due to the likelihood of experimental bias and unpersuasive placebo controls, among other things.

Are there any options besides randomized, placebo-controlled trials in evaluating CAM therapies? Unfortunately, there aren't. Some people advocate collecting large amounts of clinical data from CAM practitioners based upon the rationale that if the outcomes of enough patients are evaluated, eventually real-world answers regarding the effectiveness of these therapies will be available. This is euphemistically called "outcome research," but its logic makes no sense at all. How could the clinical data from a thousand Dr. Smiths possibly ameliorate the logical and psychological impediments that we've been examining in the last few chapters?

Others advocate using randomized, controlled trials that substitute conventional therapeutic comparison groups for placebo controls. While this strategy might control for such artifacts as natural history and the Hawthorne effect, it would actually accentuate the placebo effect. To illustrate why, let us consider a trial designed to compare acupuncture to a conventional drug that is known to reduce pain. In order to enroll participants in such a study, its investigators must still obtain informed consent via a statement such as:

> You are being asked to participate in an experimental study comparing the pain relieving effects of acupuncture with those

of a nonsteroidal anti-inflammatory drug containing ibuprofen. To be eligible to participate, you must have been diagnosed with osteoarthritis of the knee....

Who is more likely to volunteer for such a trial—people who think acupuncture is ridiculous and want to help medical science prove it, or people who believe that acupuncture may indeed relieve pain without the side effects normally attendant on most conventional drugs? People who want the opportunity to try acupuncture, or people who want to try Advil for the umpteenth time?

The simple fact is that people who volunteer to participate in a CAM trial believe (or are open to believing) that the CAM therapy being tested can help them. And since everyone in this hypothetical trial of acupuncture versus ibuprofen (needles versus pills) will know from the first day which treatment they are receiving, those participants receiving acupuncture will receive a significantly greater placebo boost than their disappointed counterparts receiving the conventional drug. Thus, if anything, such a trial will enhance the placebo effect while at the same time encouraging experimental attrition.

Which means that, if anything, we are probably worse off here than we were in the scenario represented in Tables 6.3 and 6.4, where some participants at least had some uncertainty regarding the group to which they had been assigned. In fact, because CAM trials are usually conducted by individuals who fervently believe in CAM and employ participants with the same orientation, the substitution of a conventional treatment in place of a placebo means that the placebo effect is as uncontrolled as it was in Dr. Smith's original one-group trial—which is the very type of research a patient or clinician is likely to come across when doing an Internet search for evidence related to the effectiveness of CAM therapies. And this in turn means that no amount of research employing this type of design (just as no amount of outcome data collected from CAM practitioners) will answer our original question of whether or not any CAM therapy is more effective in producing positive health outcomes than a placebo.

What are the options? There is only one I know of, and that is to consider only *high-quality* evidence relevant to the existence of CAM therapeutic effects independent of those attributable to placebos (which will help to ensure the credibility of that evidence) and then to judge the plausibility of that evidence. Before doing this, however, we need to establish some ground rules for objectively judging both the credibility and plausibility of scientific evidence.

CHAPTER SEVEN

Judging the Credibility and Plausibility of Scientific Evidence

I think everyone is aware that there is a major distinction between what is considered acceptable scientific evidence and what is considered to be appropriate legal, political, or religious evidence. I think, too, that most people understand that there are also major distinctions between what is considered to be acceptable evidence among the various scientific disciplines. Some sciences are primarily observational in nature, some are primarily experimental, and many are both.

Medicine, once commonly considered an art, is now largely evidence-driven, and the science that generates this evidence is of two sorts: biochemical experiments designed to understand *how* the body might react to a given therapy under the best of circumstances, and randomized clinical trials (RCTs) designed to ascertain *if* the body reacts to that therapy under controlled circumstances. The first genre, how or why a therapeutic effect might occur, is primarily conducted for two reasons: to help develop new therapies (primarily drugs) and to provide evidence for the plausibility of these treatments once they are subjected to RCTs. The second genre of research is designed to produce credible evidence that a therapeutic effect does actually occur in real life, and it is necessitated by the unfortunate fact that just because something is plausible (e.g., a predicted chemical reaction can be measured in a test tube, the tissues of a diseased rat, or the blood of human volunteers) does not mean that it will occur with sufficient potency in real patients to actually cure anything.

In the best of all possible worlds, it should be easy to look at both sources of evidence for each type of CAM therapy and decide whether or not there is a credible experiment demonstrating that it does work in the real world and, if it does work, whether there is a plausible scientific rationale for why it works. In fact, in a perfect world it shouldn't even be necessary to explain why something works if we're sure that indeed it does. After all, we knew that penicillin was a true wonder drug years before we knew what happened in the body to make it so effective.

But if the past few chapters have demonstrated anything, I would hope that it would be that just because someone with a Ph.D. or M.D. performs a clinical trial doesn't mean that the trial possesses any credibility whatsoever. In fact, the vast majority of these efforts are worse than worthless because they produce misleading results.

So despite the fact that there have literally been hundreds of thousands of medical experiments conducted over the past few decades, there are almost always huge gaps in this experimental record.[1] And even worse, as everyone who watches the nightly news knows, often this embarrassment of riches is accompanied by diametrically conflicting results. One week we hear that oat bran reduces serum cholesterol; the next report we see says that it does not. First we are told that estrogen replacement protects against heart disease; later we are informed that it causes it.[2]

And as bad as this situation is in conventional medicine, it is far worse in CAM. There are many CAM therapies that have never been evaluated via a randomized, placebo-controlled trial. And there are therapies that have been evaluated multiple times so poorly that some trials argue definitively for their effectiveness while others demonstrate their complete impotence. It has been estimated, in fact, that more than 500 RCTs have been conducted to evaluate acupuncture alone, half of which have been placebo-controlled, yet the number of high-quality acupuncture trials could probably be counted on one's fingers.[3] And there are precious few therapies for which *any* high-quality effectiveness evidence exists at all.

How does one go about evaluating this evidence, including its gaps and its contradictions? By evaluating both the credibility and the plausibility of that evidence.

CREDIBILITY

Credibility of evidence is evaluated by those who are well versed in judging the procedural quality of clinical trials—a task greatly facilitated by the fact that all CAM experiments are not created equally, as illustrated by the following hierarchy:

1. Randomized clinical trials are more credible than nonrandomized ones.
2. Large RCTs (those with at least fifty patients per group and preferably more than one hundred) are more credible than small ones.
3. Large double-blinded RCTs employing placebo control groups are more credible than RCTs not employing placebos, especially for CAM trials.
4. Large double-blinded randomized, placebo-controlled trials with relatively minor experimental attrition (preferably less than 20 percent but certainly less than 25 percent) are more credible than large randomized, placebo-controlled trials with high experimental attrition.
5. Large double-blinded randomized, placebo-controlled clinical trials with low attrition rates published in high-quality journals are more credible (primarily because they screen trials more stringently on both quality and credibility) than large randomized, placebo-controlled clinical trials published in, say, complementary and alternative journals that consistently have a bias favoring studies showing that CAM works.

6. Large double-blinded randomized, placebo-controlled clinical trials with low experimental attrition published in high-quality scientific journals that have been independently validated by other investigators are the most credible type of evidence available to us.

PLAUSIBILITY

The second approach to judging gaps and contradictions in the research record involves evaluating the plausibility of the experimental therapy itself. Therapies such as penicillin or insulin, whose effectiveness was so immediately obvious that clinical trials evaluating them were really superfluous, are few and far between.[4] So physiologically oriented scientists, who know full well that clinical effectiveness trials are geared toward producing false positive results (because of experimenter bias, placebo effects, regression to the mean, natural history, incomplete blinding, and a plethora of other factors), feel much more confident about a therapy if there is basic research (involving tissue samples or rats that can be dissected) that predicts that the therapy *should* work before the trial is even conceived.

Medicine (an applied science that encompasses biology, physiology, pharmacology, biochemistry, genetics, and a host of other basic sciences) has now reached a point where the biochemical mechanisms for just about all of its more effective therapies are understood. The discipline is so heavily reliant upon explaining these biochemical mechanisms, in fact, that it is practically unheard of for a major clinical trial to be conducted involving a treatment for which there is not an already known biochemical mechanism capable of explaining why a specific health outcome should occur.[5] If funding for conducting a trial were somehow to be obtained and the resulting effort produced results that had no credible biochemical explanation, many scientists would actually discount these findings until either additional evidence was produced and became so overwhelming that the phenomenon could not be sensibly ignored or a plausible physiological mechanism was discovered.

While this insistence upon understanding the why of things may seem a bit anal, in many ways it is logically defensible. If, for example, we know for a fact that drug A contains chemical B, which is known to suppress toxin C in tissue samples taken from exposed animals, and if we know from other research that the presence of toxin C is associated with symptom D (as determined by either human or animal studies), then a positive clinical trial finding that drug A does relieve symptom D is simply a lot more believable than if drug A were the brainchild of a mad chemist who mixed a few ingredients in his laboratory and then conducted a clinical trial to evaluate it.

Now, of course the credibility (quality) of these preliminary animal studies is just as important as is the credibility of the human RCTs we've been discussing. The problem is that they involve completely different quality criteria (e.g., the typical animal study is conducted with six to eight animals per group and almost never as many as fifty), and the reporting of what goes on in animal studies is much less detailed than is the case for large RCTs. (It is interesting to note, however, that placebo groups are routinely employed in this type of research, such as by injecting one group of animals with a saline solution in order to compare their response with those injected with a drug.) Animal experiments are also much cheaper to conduct (once an investigator has an established laboratory), so they can be run more easily and more frequently, and if something goes wrong, the whole thing can be scrapped and the investigators can start all over again. Since these studies can be mounted rather quickly and conducted rather cheaply, however, important findings (such as chemical B suppressing toxin C in rat tissues) that emerge from animal studies are much more likely than those emerging from RCTs to be replicated both by the original investigators themselves and by other labs.

Judging the plausibility of CAM research is just as important as it is for conventional findings, but CAM is at somewhat of a disadvantage because its proposed mechanisms of action often do not involve known physiological systems. Still, if a positive analgesic effect for acupuncture is obtained in an RCT, then the plausibility of that effect will be greatly enhanced if there is supporting biochemical research that can explain the how or why of it. But if the primary biochemical explanation for how these little needles reduce pain involves an unmeasurable energy force surging through some unobservable meridians with no documented connection to pain or anything else, then most members of the scientific community will have a difficult time believing these positive results, even if they're from an otherwise credible clinical trial (e.g., a trial of sufficient size that employs a credible randomized placebo control group).

If acupuncture worked as dramatically as penicillin, then we could totally ignore the annoying biologists. If, on the other hand, acupuncture worked only as dramatically as a placebo, then the therapy's proponents would have somewhat of a scientific public relations problem on their hands.

Thus our purpose in examining both the plausibility and the credibility of the existing scientific record surrounding the CAM-placebo dyad is directed toward providing an educated choice between two options: whether the pain reduction benefits derivable from therapies such as acupuncture are specific to these therapies or can be attributable to placebo (or placebo-like) effects.

None of this will be relevant to people whose beliefs are more important to them than whether or not those beliefs are correct. Discussions such as this are relevant only for those individuals who are willing to consider the possibility that science represents a reasonable path toward providing specific answers to exceedingly specific questions— people, in other words, who believe that science has its place in the world of thought and that one of those places is in the protection, restoration, and maintenance of our health.

THE PLAN OF ATTACK

For the enlightenment of this latter group of readers, I therefore propose in the remainder of this book to examine four types of evidence. First, in order to ascertain if those effects attributable to CAM therapies are

indeed placebo effects, I will examine the credibility of the evidence surrounding the issue of whether there is even such a thing as a placebo effect. Second, since plausibility in medical science is so closely associated with biochemical changes that occur within the body, I will discuss the evidence regarding whether placebos have ever been demonstrated to effect such changes.

Next (assuming that some of this evidence is promising as far as the placebo effect is concerned), I will do the same thing for CAM therapies—that is, examine whether there is any credible evidence out there that a CAM therapy has been shown to be more effective than a placebo. And finally, I will examine the plausibility of the biochemical rationales currently proposed to explain why CAM therapies *should* produce analgesic effects.

In the best of all possible worlds, these four types of evidence should provide simple yes-or-no answers to the following four questions:

1. Is there such a thing as a therapeutic placebo effect?
2. Is there a plausible biochemical analgesic mechanism of action that could explain such an effect?
3. Is there such a thing as a CAM therapeutic effect over and above what can be attributed to the placebo effect (assuming that there is such a thing as the latter)?
4. Are there plausible biochemical mechanisms of action that could explain these CAM therapeutic effects (assuming there are such things)?

What happens if less-than-definitive answers are provided to these questions in our all-too-imperfect world? All will not be lost, since we can always lean upon a principle that scientists themselves have been using for centuries to choose between competing theories in the presence of less than definitive research evidence: the parsimony principle.

THE PARSIMONY PRINCIPLE

In science there are always an infinite number of possible explanations for the occurrence of any phenomenon, which is why we conduct research in the first place—to weed out as many of these alternative explanations as possible. But what happens when this research falls flat on its face or hasn't even been conducted?

The answer may surprise you: we fall back upon advice of a Catholic monk who lived over half a millennium ago. In the fourteenth century the scientific philosopher William of Occam advanced a now almost universally accepted "rule of evidence" for choosing between two (or more) rival explanations, either in the absence of adequate data or when the data appear to support both theories equally well. Known as Occam's razor (because it was designed to cut directly through irrelevancies and straight to the bone) or the parsimony principle, this rule was succinctly phrased by its originator as follows: "What is done with fewer assumptions is done in vain with more." Note that William of Occam was too astute to use words such as *plausibility* or *credibility*. He simply counseled us to accept the theory that required the fewest unproven assumptions.

Thus, since at this point in our journey we have presented no real evidence one way or another regarding the biochemical mechanism for either CAM therapies or the placebo effect, Occam's razor could easily be applied to my thesis that the two are one and the same phenomenon. As an example, let's consider the plausibility of two of the most commonly advanced explanations for why people who receive acupuncture to relieve knee pain often actually do report improvement following its receipt.

Explanation 1: The reduction in pain following the insertion of tiny needles in the body is due to those needles modulating the flow of a type of energy (qi) through meridians that are specifically designed for this purpose (somewhat similar to the role of arteries in blood flow), thereby reducing the subject's pain.

Explanation 2: The reduction in pain following the insertion of tiny little needles in the body is due to the placebo effect, which is a phenomenon hypothesized to occur whenever a patient receives any therapy (effective or otherwise) that he or she believes will be beneficial.

Either explanation could be true, and there are a number of ways that we could choose between them. In politics, we could conduct a poll or allow our elected representatives to vote on them. If this were a religious issue, we could allow our clergy or our religious tenets to point us toward the truth. In science, we employ Occam's razor.

Now, of course, if there is *some* evidence relevant to weighing the plausibility of explanation 1 versus explanation 2, any rational individual would attempt to weigh this evidence before attempting to choose between them. However, if there really isn't any acceptable evidence available for choosing between these two explanations, then Occam's razor can always be applied.

In the present case, its application would end the debate pretty quickly. We could follow William's lead and simply count up the number of unsupported assumptions. For the first explanation, we must assume (1) the existence of an unmeasured energy form called qi, (2) an as yet undetected system of meridians through which this qi flows, (3) that the acupuncture needles are in fact capable of affecting this flow, and (4) that this altered flow is capable of reducing pain.

The second explanation requires us to assume (1) that a ceremony (of inserting tiny needles into the body accompanied by promises that such practices have reduced pain for thousands of years) can engender psychological expectations of benefit and (2) that these psychological expectations (or suggestions) can influence our perceptions of the pain we experience (or cause us to imagine that we were experiencing less pain than we really were). According to my scorecard, explanation 2 requires fewer unfounded assumptions; ergo, explanation 2 is the correct choice. And if Chapters 8 and 9 of this book are able to definitively show that there is credible evidence for the existence of such a thing as an analgesic placebo effect, and if Chapter 10 is able to buttress this inference via a plausible biochemical rationale for how this effect manifests itself, then our scorecard will be even more one-sided.

BUT IF IGNORANCE REALLY IS BLISS, WHY CAN'T WE JUST BE HAPPY?

Just because I am a scientist and, as such, believe in *evidence* doesn't mean that everyone else has to. And just because I happen to believe that the knowledge this evidence generates is ultimately beneficial to us (regardless of whether it is always pleasing) and that in the long run we are better off operating from a position of knowledge than from one of ignorance doesn't mean that I am correct. Whatever my own views and whatever the value I place on scientific evidence, an eminently reasonable question remains:

> If complementary and alternative therapies do make people feel better, is it important for people to know that the therapies do this for the wrong reason?

Having such knowledge is seldom of lifesaving significance. Sugar pills are not harmful to anyone other than diabetics, and a passing understanding of the logical, statistical, and emotional reasoning artifacts that *may* encourage people to pay others to stick little needles into their bodies or to manipulate their spinal columns is not a major survival skill.

True, there are CAM proponents out there who irresponsibly attempt to sell CAM therapies en masse to an unsuspecting public. In reviewing the recommendations made by the authors of seven popular CAM books, for example, Edzard Ernst and colleagues found that on average 73 different CAM therapies were favorably mentioned for each of thirty-five different medical conditions, with cancer having 133 separate CAM recommendations.[6]

But it is also true that CAM charlatans are probably more of an irritant than a cause for alarm. While the public can be gullible at times, it is not stupid. In an analysis of a national survey, two colleagues and I found that very few individuals nationwide seek CAM therapies for serious diseases such as cancer or heart disease and hardly anyone does so in lieu of conventional medical care.[7] Occasionally a high-profile individual such as Coretta Scott King goes to a CAM treatment center for the treatment of a life-threatening disease (she went to the same center that prescribed laetrile to Steve McQueen just before *his* death), but such events are rare and probably occur primarily as a last resort.

So if the issues involved here are generally *not* that crucial, why have I inflicted them upon my unsuspecting public? I suppose it is partly due to an admittedly irritating tendency to instruct (which I lay at the doorstep of my parents, who were teachers before me). And partly it is due to a common professional objective for a scientist: to be able to claim a personal victory in one small skirmish in the perpetual struggle between knowledge and ignorance.

Even a tiny skirmish such as this necessitates a journey through different layers of a body of scientific evidence that has never really been mapped in any systematic, accessible way. Indeed, it is the description of this journey, and the accompanying process of weighing evidence from some very disparate sources, that this book promised a while back to undertake. Now is the time for it to do just that—to take you, my readers, to the border separating what is known about placebo effects and CAM therapies from what is yet to be discovered, and to let you decide for yourselves if you agree or disagree with my interpretation of what appears to be on both sides of this boundary.

CHAPTER EIGHT

Some Personal Research Involving Acupuncture

Of the various impediments to interpreting the results of randomized, controlled trials of complementary and alternative medical therapies, the most problematic involves the difficulties involved in constructing credible placebo controls. In this chapter I will illustrate the importance of this issue via some research in which I was personally involved during my tenure with the University of Maryland's NIH-funded Complementary Medicine Program.

I believe that describing this firsthand experience is crucial as a point of reference for the remainder of the book, in which I will primarily discuss placebo and CAM research conducted by other investigators. There is always a leap of faith taken when reviewing the work of others. For one thing, it is necessary to assume that what they report about their investigations is exactly what was done in the actual trials. In addition, one has to assume that they have duly reported any serious problems arising during the course of a trial, even though for too many researchers the difficulty of doing so is akin to a camel traversing the eye of a needle—a problem that is compounded by the fact that a surprisingly large number of principal investigators are not integrally involved with what goes on during their trials but rely on other people to run the studies for them. Either way, whether they write the research reports themselves or rely upon someone else to do that for them as well, it is very tempting to simply not mention little glitches that occurred during the course of the studies. Or, depending upon the situation, it can be equally tempting for the person who did do the work not to report these little glitches to his or her boss.

So, in truth, I won't be able to swear to the validity of any of the other studies that I will review in the next few chapters, although a number of the laboratory experiments involved in demonstrating the existence of the placebo effect and its physiological mechanism (at least for pain) have been replicated by other researchers. While I will effuse about the placebo mechanism experiments conducted by such scientists as Fabrizio Benedetti, Martina Amanzio, Antonella Pollo, and colleagues—and while I have corresponded with Fabrizio Benedetti several times and published his work in the journal I have edited for many years, *Evaluation and the Health Professions*—I have not observed any of these researchers at work, nor have I even met any of them personally. The same is true for the research conducted by Donald Price and others that I will so admiringly describe.

I do, however, have firsthand experience with respect to acupuncture efficacy trials, having personally supervised the conduct of several, and hence can attest to what happened during their conduct. Fortuitously, two of these trials were designed to help ameliorate the failing that so bedevils CAM research: the credibility of its placebos.

ACUPUNCTURE FOR PAIN DUE TO DENTAL SURGERY

The rationale for these two studies[1] was based on an article that analyzed sixteen trials conducted over a twenty-year period on the effectiveness of acupuncture in treating acute dental pain. The authors of the review, with the appropriate disclaimers, concluded: "On balance, these data suggest that acupuncture is effective in alleviating pain either during dental operations, following surgery or during experimentally induced dental pain in human volunteers."[2] (I'll discuss the nature of systematic reviews themselves in greater depth in Chapter 12; for now, it's worth noting that, as of a few years ago, at least thirty-nine systematic reviews have been conducted to address the use of acupuncture for a wide range of medical conditions, including chronic pain, asthma, drug addiction, nausea, and vomiting.[3] The most common outcome variable employed was, of course, pain relief. While some of these reviews are redundant, at least thirty are not.[4])

Some researchers took immediate and serious issue with the article's conclusion, citing such concerns as the lack of randomization, small sample sizes, and the absence of effective placebo controls, but nevertheless the bottom-line conclusion of the review was that acupuncture was effective.[5] To the authors' credit, however, they did mention that when assessed on the 5-point Jadad quality scale, none of the sixteen studies reviewed scored higher than a 3 (which is considered barely adequate), and five (31 percent) actually (and incredibly) scored zero—which illustrates what is *really* the most serious issue involved in interpreting CAM research: so much of it appears to totally disregard (or to be totally ignorant of) methodological quality.[6] This abysmal lack of research quality makes interpreting the results of any CAM systematic review extremely difficult.

Regardless, the trials were conducted and published, and the systematic review of them was performed and published. And in the reviewers' defense, they did supplement their positive conclusion about acupuncture by acknowledging the importance of the placebo effect in interpreting the results of CAM research:

> The placebo effect of acupuncture as a treatment for pain can be impressive; this is shown convincingly in one randomized, double-blind trial [which the authors cite] in which the majority of patients treated with sham acupuncture responded with significant pain relief.[7]

Given how "impressive" the placebo effect truly is, is it any wonder that most CAM therapists honestly do believe that they are helping people? And is it at all surprising that most CAM patients truly believe that they are being helped? Finally, is it any wonder that so many researchers can be hoodwinked as well?

But if there is a silver lining in this cloud of abysmally conducted acupuncture trials, it is the fact that it generated research that provided a definitive answer to the question of whether acupuncture is capable of relieving acute dental pain (in this case pain following dental surgery) over and above what can be attributed to the placebo effect. Thanks to Dr. Lixing Lao, I was able to participate in producing this answer via a pair of randomized, placebo-controlled trials. (Lao, incidentally, in addition to having been trained as a traditional Chinese medical doctor at the Shanghai University of Traditional Chinese Medicine, has a Ph.D. in physiology from the University of Maryland, is an associate professor at the University of Maryland School of Medicine, and also was on the faculty of the Maryland Institute of Traditional Chinese Medicine for ten years.)

The first trial consisted of evaluating whether or not acupuncture could exert an analgesic effect over and above the use of a local anesthetic following a tooth extraction (in this case, a partially impacted wisdom tooth). One hundred and twenty patients were randomly assigned to one of three groups: an experimental group consisting of those receiving real acupuncture and two placebo groups. Indeed, one of Lao's primary goals in conducting this study, and one of the reasons that the NIH funded it in the first place, was that he wanted to develop the "perfect" placebo control group for use by future acupuncture researchers. A "perfect" placebo should possess two equally important characteristics: the people who are assigned to receive it should not be able to distinguish it from the real therapy being assessed, and it must have no active therapeutic effect of its own. With this in mind, Lao designed his acupuncture and placebo (or fake) acupuncture experiences to be as identical as humanly possible. The true acupuncture procedure employed the insertion of needles to a depth of 0.3 to 0.5 inches into four points based upon traditional Chinese medicine: three in the face and one in the hand, with a piece of tape placed next to each needle. To help keep the participants from knowing whether they were receiving real or fake acupuncture, a fake insertion was made in the knee, which was accomplished by using the edge of the needle's guide tube to elicit a sensation, after which an acupuncture needle was taped, but not inserted, at the point of contact. (While this location may appear odd, classic Chinese meridian theory sometimes uses locations in the body that are completely removed from the location of the pain.)

Patients in the two placebo groups both received exactly the same number of acupuncture points as the real procedure. The first placebo group received a sham (fake) noninsertion at the same four classic acupuncture points used in the true acupuncture group, accompanied by one shallow insertion (0.1 to 0.3 inches) at a nonactive point in the knee. (This shallow insertion was effected in the classic mode, but not as deeply.) The second placebo group received a shallow insertion at the four non-acupuncture points and one sham noninsertion at the same nonactive knee point used in the other two groups.

All participants' eyes were covered so that they could not observe any of the procedures, true or sham, while they were occurring. In all three groups, inserted needles were twisted manually three times as follows: during initial insertion, at the midpoint of the twenty-minute treatment, and at the end of the treatment session in order to elicit what traditional Chinese practitioners call *de qi*.[8] For the noninserted needles, the guide tube was used to simulate this twisting mechanism. While no electrical current was applied to any patient in the study (true or sham), one further attempt was made to trick the patients by using a mock electrical stimulation unit in all three groups. This unit was equipped with a blinking light and a ticking sound. Patients were told that they might or might not feel the electrical current because of the nature of the device. And, just to be safe, we didn't allow anyone who had previously experienced acupuncture to participate in the trial.

The results were quite definitive: *there was no statistically significant difference between the real acupuncture group and the two placebo groups with respect to the average pain experienced following dental surgery.*

But then came the truly unusual aspect of this study. As part of his design, Lao had convinced the NIH to allow him to conduct a second trial that would be identical to the first except that it would be larger and would substitute another placebo acupuncture procedure for the least promising placebo group employed in the original trial. In other words, it would be an identical replication for the real acupuncture procedure and *one* of the placebo procedures.

Thus, we repeated the first trial with a larger sample (180 patients) and substituted a different placebo control group for the second one described above. The new placebo procedure employed five acupuncture points adjacent to the classical points, but all used the sham noninsertion technique. The results of the second experiment were identical to those of the first: there was no difference between real and fake acupuncture with respect to the average amount of pain experienced or the time it took for the patients local analgesia to wear off. (As expected, none of the placebo procedures differed from one another with respect to pain relief either.)

Table 8.1 summarizes these results, both individually and for all of the data combined—which was reasonable, since both trials' procedures were so similar.

While it is undoubtedly immodest of me to say this, it should be noted that these two trials were of extremely high quality for CAM research. They employed sufficiently large numbers of patients (combined, they included a total of 100 patients per group and averaged 150 per group for the comparisons of the experimental variable and the combined placebos), and they employed not one but a total of three placebo groups. Equally rare in CAM research, experimental attrition (i.e., participants dropping out of the study before it was completed) was almost nonexistent in these trials: no participants dropped out of the first trial, and only three (2 percent) dropped out of the second (because we had to let them go home early due to a snowstorm). Still, like all acupuncture trials, we couldn't report that our studies were completely double-blinded. We took pains to blind the patients, the research assistants who collected data from them, and even the esteemed biostatistician who

Table 8.1. Effects of Acupuncture on Postoperative Dental Pain

	True Acupuncture (Experimental)		Placebo Acupuncture (Combined Controls)		Statistical Significance
	Mean (95% CI)**	N	Mean (95% CI)	N	
Experiment 1					
Mean of pain VAS,* 1st to 2nd treatment	24.1 (18.3–29.9)	40	24.9 (20.2–29.6)	80	Not statistically significant
Experiment 2					
Mean of pain VAS, 1st to 2nd treatment	24.7 (19.6–29.8)	60	28.7 (24.3–33.2)	120	Not statistically significant
Experiments 1 and 2 combined					
Mean of pain VAS, 1st to 2nd treatment	24.5 (20.7–28.2)	100	27.2 (24.0–30.5)	200	Not statistically significant

* VAS = visual analog scale

** CI = confidence interval, a statistical representation of the range in which a group mean can vary due to chance alone.

analyzed the data according to random codes to prevent his knowing which group was which. We also attempted to control the acupuncturists' behavior by writing a script for them to follow that was designed to minimize any verbal hints they might give away to patients regarding group membership. That said, the acupuncturists still knew which patients were received the "real" treatment and which were receiving a placebo. This meant that, like all acupuncture trials, our acupuncture groups probably received an additional placebo boost from the acupuncturists themselves.

Normally the story would end here, but these two experiments produced something besides their negative findings, which was a completely unexpected result that shocked both Lao and me.

THE SURPRISE

While he had tested the credibility of his placebo procedures with a few test cases prior to conducting the actual trials, Lao did something that all investigators (CAM and conventional) should do but seldom bother with: he instituted a check to see if his placebo groups really did indeed trick people. This blinding check consisted of a single question, which was asked of both the real acupuncture group and the two placebo groups.

Question:
Which treatment do you *think* you received?

Responses:
a. Real acupuncture
b. Fake acupuncture
c. Not sure

This simple question was asked three times during the course of the trial: (1) just after the participants' first acupuncture treatment, (2) when (and if) a participant reported experiencing moderate to severe pain (at which point the participant received a second real or placebo acupuncture treatment, depending upon the group to which the participant had been randomly assigned), and (3) at the end of the six-hour period (which constituted the entire trial).

Table 8.2 indicates what we found immediately after the first acupuncture treatment, namely, that the fake acupuncture procedures were fairly good at tricking their recipients. Almost a third of the patients (30.5 percent) in these two groups believed that they were receiving the real thing, another 50 percent were uncertain which treatment they

Table 8.2. Combined Results for Patient Beliefs Regarding Group Membership (Blinding Success)

	Patients Who Believed They Were Receiving True Acupuncture	Patients Who Were Unsure Which Treatment They Were Receiving	Patients Who Believed They Were Receiving One of the Placebo Treatments
	N (%)	*N* (%)	*N* (%)
Patients actually receiving real acupuncture	43 (43.0%)	53 (53.0%)	4 (4.0%)
Patients actually receiving the placebo	61 (30.5%)	100 (50.0%)	39 (19.5%)

were receiving, and 19.5 percent of the patients in the placebo groups were convinced that they were receiving a placebo.

Meanwhile, the patients in the real acupuncture group were more likely to correctly guess that they were receiving real acupuncture (43 percent), which probably explains why these patients reported slightly (but not statistically significant) less pain than did the patients in the placebo group. Still, 57 percent of even the acupuncture patients either were unsure or thought they were receiving the placebo procedure; hence the blinding procedures were *fairly* effective for these participants as well.

In effect, then, this means that the overall trial results were even more negative than Table 8.1 indicates. Why? Because the real acupuncture groups should have received an additional placebo boost over and above the sham acupuncture groups based upon the fact that more of the participants in the real acupuncture groups believed they were receiving something beneficial than was the case for the participants in the placebo groups. These differences weren't that dramatic, however, and since some patients often figure out which group they are in by the end of most trials, CAM or non-CAM, this was *not* the finding that surprised us.[9]

By delving a little deeper into the data (which is what people like me do on the weekends while our peers are mowing the lawn or shoveling snow), your venerable author found the following interesting little tidbit: while acupuncture didn't do anything for the participants' pain (at least in contrast to the placebos), those patients who believed (as shown in Table 8.3) that they were getting real acupuncture experienced significantly less pain than those who believed that they were getting fake acupuncture. And this held true regardless of whether they were receiving the real thing or the placebo, and it held true for both experiments.

In some ways this difference is easier to visualize graphically. Thus when the difference in pain between patients who received real acupuncture versus placebo acupuncture (from Table 8.1) are graphed against those who thought they were receiving real acupuncture versus those who thought they were receiving the placebo (Table 8.3), a truly dramatic pattern emerges, as shown in Figure 8.1.

Table 8.3. Effects of Patient Belief upon Pain

	Patients Who Believed They Were Receiving True Acupuncture		Patients Who Were Unsure Which Treatment They Were Receiving		Patients Who Believed They Were Receiving One of the Placebo Treatments		Statistical Significance
	Mean (95% CI)	N	Mean (95% CI)	N	Mean (95% CI)	N	
Experiment 1							
Mean of pain VAS,* 1st to 2nd treatment	17.5 (13.6–21.3)	31	24.7 (20.1–29.3)	71	36.8 (22.6–51.0)	18	Yes
Experiment 2							
Mean of pain VAS, 1st to 2nd treatment	22.5 (17.3–27.6)	73	27.0 (22.5–31.5)	82	42.9 (31.7–54.1)	25	Yes
Combined experiments							
Mean of pain VAS, 1st to 2nd treatment	21.0 (17.2–24.8)	104	26.0 (22.8–29.2)	153	40.4 (31.9–48.8)	43	Yes

* VAS = visual analog scale

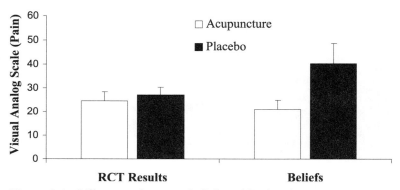

Figure 8.1. Differences Between Beliefs and Reality: Acupuncture versus Placebo Effects upon Pain

I should mention straight off that the results in Figure 8.1 do not categorically demonstrate that the placebo effect is stronger than acupuncture effects or that acupuncture effects are synonymous with placebo effects. They don't even necessarily represent cause and effect. (Of course, the statistically insignificant difference between the acupuncture and the placebo groups is causal in nature because patients were randomly assigned to these groups.) Nevertheless, consider the following two alternative explanations for the results.

Alternative explanation 1: beliefs regarding group membership caused the differences in pain relief (or perceptions of pain relief, which is pretty much the same thing). While this may well be true, unfortunately our trials were designed to test cause and effect only for acupuncture effects, not belief. To ascertain causation, it would be necessary to experimentally manipulate beliefs. This is certainly possible, as will be illustrated in the next chapter's discussion of patients who are tricked into thinking they are receiving a real therapy when all they are getting is a placebo, but we didn't do that in our own trials.

Alternative explanation 2: differences in pain caused (or influenced) differences in patients' guesses regarding which treatment they were receiving. In other words, at the point in time when first asked which treatment they thought they were receiving, some patients were simply experiencing more pain than others. People are different, after all. And since almost everyone who volunteers for an acupuncture trial believes that acupuncture can relieve pain, those participants who were experiencing more pain than they had expected might very well assume that they were not receiving acupuncture. The opposite is true as well: those people whose pain wasn't too bad (due to either the local anesthetic or the placebo effect) might have incorrectly attributed this low level of pain to acupuncture.

I would like to think that it was our participants' beliefs that triggered a placebo effect that in turn actually resulted in decreased pain (alternative explanation 1). But in the final analysis, it doesn't much matter what the "real" explanation for these results is since we know that patients didn't make their guesses based upon the effects of acupuncture. Why? *Because there weren't any effects for acupuncture.* The participants made their guesses based upon their personal beliefs and expectations, which is the essence of what we've been talking about for more than a hundred pages now.

Thus what we have here is another illustration of the role of expectations and beliefs in people's personal evaluations of whether or not a CAM therapy helped them. This relationship can be summed up as follows: If we believe in CAM therapies, then they will most likely work for us. If they don't work for us, then we will find a reason for this failure and continue to believe in them—thereby prohibiting reality from conflicting with our beliefs.

There was a unique aspect to these findings:

They provided a direct comparison of the expectations of CAM effectiveness versus actual CAM effectiveness. And the results weren't even close!

This conundrum once again epitomizes the difficulties that people have in making inferences based upon their personal experiences. It also provides one additional illustration of why scientists find it so difficult to remain objective and why so much of the evidence they produce is influenced by their personal beliefs and expectations. Finally, on a more mundane level, it also illustrates why it can be so difficult to answer a straightforward, simple question such as "Are CAM therapies more effective than placebos?" and also why hardly anyone will believe such an answer once it is generated unless they happened to start out with that opinion. Ultimately, however, I am pleased to report that Agent Mulder was absolutely correct all along: the truth is "out there"—it is just a bit difficult for people to accept. And it is upon the search for that truth that we are now ready to embark.

CHAPTER NINE

How We Know That the Placebo Effect Exists

It is time to begin the process of weighing and evaluating evidence because of one simple fact: *people often do feel better after they have received a complementary and alternative therapy.* This, in turn, requires us to choose between the two most popular rival hypotheses, beliefs, explanations, or opinions (take your pick) advanced for explaining this strange fact: (1) CAM recipients feel better because of some biochemical, energetic, magical, or unknown component of the therapies themselves, or (2) CAM recipients feel better because of the placebo effect.

While these two hypotheses are diametrically opposed to each other, definitively demonstrating that one is categorically false and the other is categorically true is difficult because of the number of CAM therapies involved, the fact that most of them have not been studied under carefully controlled conditions, and the conflicting conclusions that have resulted from those therapies that have been studied. But like it or not, that is exactly where we are at this point and where we are heading—facing the necessity of choosing between two hypotheses in the presence of imperfect evidence. Welcome to the wonderful world of science!

Fortunately, while the evidence may be imperfect, there is enough of it out there for us to avoid falling back on William of Occam's razor—but only after the evidence is weighed very carefully. What I propose to do in this chapter, therefore, is to explore the evidence surrounding the existence of the placebo effect in sufficient detail to answer the following question:

Is there really such a thing as an analgesic placebo effect?

WHY PROVE THE OBVIOUS?

One of the primary functions of science is to provide an objective, number-driven method to decide which of two positions is most likely to be correct, because we learned a long time ago that we can't simply poll scientists, CAM therapists, or anyone else in order to allow the majority to provide the answer. If this were done, at any given point in history for any given scientific hypothesis the majority opinion would have been more likely to be wrong than right. Before Copernicus, a vote by the best and brightest minds would have definitively placed the earth at the center of the universe. Before Einstein, 99 percent of the scientific community would have considered time and space to be as immutable as a piece of granite. And as illustrated by a quotation from a speech given by nineteenth-century physicist James Clerk Maxwell—greatly admired by Einstein, incidentally—the process of conversion from one theory to another is a bit short of instantaneous: "There are two theories of the nature of light, the corpuscle theory and the wave theory; we used to believe in the corpuscle theory; now we believe in the wave theory because all who believed in the corpuscle theory have died."[1]

Since none of us has time to wait for such a major die-off, a scientist's only option when faced with two conflicting hypotheses is to build the best possible case for one or the other theory based upon the best possible evidence and to do so without falling back upon unproven assumptions. Thus the short answer to why we need to prove the obvious is that in science, unproven assumptions, even "obvious" ones, should be avoided like the plague. Failing this, we must face William of Occam's relentless blade, which to a scientist is most unpalatable (and unsatisfying for everyone else).

CREDIBILITY REVISITED, OR WHO GETS TO DECIDE WHAT THE "BEST EVIDENCE" IS?

We discussed some of the criteria for judging the credibility of research in Chapter 7—criteria, it will be remembered, that were necessitated by several unfortunate facts of life:

1. Some scientific studies are not adequately performed because their investigators are not as competent (or as conscientious) as others.

2. Some studies are not honestly reported because some investigators are not as ethical as others. (Which means, in turn, that we can't always be sure that what the investigators said was performed or that all of the study's limitations and mistakes were mentioned.)

3. Some investigators allow their biases to influence their results.

All of which leads us to the point where we now find ourselves in CAM research: in possession of an unorganized body of conflicting evidence supporting and not supporting the effectiveness of this or that treatment. And while any competent biostatistician can look at the written report of a clinical trial and judge whether or not it was adequately designed and executed (judging by factors such as the presence or absence of a placebo control group, as discussed in Chapter 7), even the best of us can't be sure that what is reported was actually done, that all of the study limitations (and mistakes) have been reported, whether the investigators allowed their biases to influence their results, and—most important from a bottom-line perspective—whether the results reported are valid.

So how do we get around these problems? By requiring the independent confirmation of important findings, which is really the best (but not infallible) way to weed out experimenter bias and perhaps to unearth or redress unreported flaws in the original research. Hence independent confirmation is the litmus test for all important scientific discoveries. No experienced scientist, for example, is likely to accept at face value a single experiment breathlessly announcing the development of a technique for producing cold fusion or the long-awaited cure for cancer until other scientists have replicated these results.

Unfortunately, in both CAM and placebo research, independent replication is relatively rare, so for this reason we can't really apply this criterion to either area in the chapters that follow. Fortunately, there has been a considerable amount of independent verification in the laboratory (i.e., in research that uses healthy participants as opposed to patients suffering from actual medical conditions) involving the relief of pain, so I will concentrate upon that condition in both this and the next chapter, which are dedicated simply to ascertaining if a placebo effect exists and, if so, what causes it.

Before presenting the direct high-quality evidence supporting the existence of the placebo effect for pain, however, I would like to describe some indirect evidence in order to provide a historical gestalt of placebo research in general.

INDIRECT EVIDENCE THAT THE PLACEBO EFFECT EXISTS

One possible (and exceedingly simple) explanation for the placebo effect, especially for something as personal and subjective as pain, would be that the effect is entirely in the recipient's mind. On one level our working definition of a placebo actually implies such an explanation (i.e., an inactive substance can have a therapeutic effect if administered to a patient who believes that he or she is receiving an effective treatment), which in turn implies that the therapeutic effect itself, generated as it is by an inactive "treatment," may be not real but only imagined.

There happens to be some indirect evidence, however, that while the placebo effect may indeed be in our minds, it is not a figment of our imaginations. This evidence comes from someone whose name is very recognizable to most of us: Ivan Petrovich Pavlov, whose seminal contribution to science, classical conditioning, is hypothesized to be the primary triggering mechanism for the placebo effect. Arguably the most important psychophysiological finding of the nineteenth and twentieth centuries, it is highly unlikely that conditioning is a function of the imagination. Because Pavlov studied dogs, he was forced to rely upon their physiological responses rather than the human self-reports so often employed in both CAM and placebo research. So let's review what Pavlov (and some of his successors) did that is so relevant to the placebo effect. In so doing I am going to rely upon an excellent book chapter written by Shepard Siegel, a professor of psychology, on the topic.[2]

In studying the physiology of canine digestion, Pavlov learned that secretion of gastric acids in the stomach (which is a reflex not directly under the dogs' control) could eventually be triggered not only by the presence of food but also by the appearance of the individual who brought the food—even when this person arrived with no food in hand. Thus the original stimulus started out as food and the response was the secretion of stomach acid. After enough trials, the research assistants inadvertently became the stimulus because the dogs started to secrete stomach acid every time the assistants came in the room. Later, for the sake of convenience, Pavlov switched to salivation as his response (also a reflex but one whose observation doesn't require surgical access to the interior of a dog's stomach) in lieu of gastric secretions. He also switched to other stimuli, such as a specific tone or buzzer—perhaps to avoid wear and tear on his research assistants' running back and forth with food trays. What he was able to demonstrate very convincingly was that after the sound had been paired with food enough times, the sound itself could elicit salivation almost 100 percent of the time in the absence of food.

Interestingly, another set of experiments using this paradigm (but performed a decade or so later by other investigators) exploited the fact that dogs naturally salivate after receiving morphine, just as they do from the sight of food. After a few morphine injections, the dogs became conditioned to the needle itself and salivated from any injection, morphine or not. If this sounds relevant to a placebo effect, it should, since a hypodermic injection of an inert substance such as saltwater is a classic placebo.

What made Pavlov's work so exciting in the early twentieth century was its implications for how we learn things. What made it so relevant to the placebo effect (although as far as I know Pavlov never mentioned the term in any of his work) was subsequent research that applied these conditioned responses to medications (and other physiological responses) that we would normally neither associate with learning nor consider to be under an organism's conscious control. In truth, however, the placebo effect is something that must be learned before it can manifest itself. And regardless of whether or not experience really is the best teacher, the name of the teacher that oversees our learning the placebo effect is *classical conditioning*.

Placebo Effects Illustrated by Conditioned Drug Effects in Humans

While the evidence isn't definitive enough to be presented in support of our main thesis here (primarily because, to my knowledge, the individual studies haven't been independently replicated), there is a considerable amount of research that demonstrates that humans can be conditioned, just as Pavlov's successors did with dogs, to respond to placebos through repeated administrations of active drugs. In one study using healthy women, for example, two researchers administered nitroglycerin in distinctively flavored tablets over the course of several weeks. Then, following the administration of the same flavored pill without nitroglycerin (i.e., a placebo pill), a change in heart rate similar to (but less dramatic than) the response for nitroglycerin was observed.[3]

Similarly, humans apparently will respond physiologically to placebos they think are caffeine, nicotine, alcohol, and a wide variety of drugs (e.g., interferon, bronchodilators and bronchoconstrictors, stimulants and sedatives, and chemotherapeutic agents) via conditioning based upon their past experiences with those substances.[4] What makes this research interesting is that in many cases the outcomes are not normally considered to be under people's control—suggesting that the placebo effect is not just a figment of the subject's imagination. Another interesting characteristic of this research is the commonsense finding that *the conditioned responses to the placebo drugs, while substantial, are almost never as strong as the initial responses to the real drug itself.* This is, in my opinion, an important finding, one to which we will refer to several times later on.

There is an apparent exception to the rule, however, and I believe a brief digression is in order here to discuss it, partly because the concept of conditioning is so integral to the placebo effect and partly because it can be a bit more involved than one would expect when applied to the types of physiological responses that we will be discussing in the next few chapters. Early on in drug conditioning research, for example, it appeared that occasionally the conditioned responses to medications occurred in the opposite direction to a drug's designed effect. From a scientific perspective this was potentially a serious finding, because in science exceptions don't prove the rule—they destroy the theory. Fortunately, these apparent exceptions arose from a misunderstanding of what constitutes a conditioned response.

As Siegel discusses in his excellent review, researchers hypothesized that if glucose were to be repeatedly injected into an organism, one would expect a rise in the organism's blood sugar due to the action of the "drug" (glucose) itself, and this did indeed occur. Then, assuming that this physiological response (the rise in blood sugar) could be conditioned, one would expect that if the glucose injections were replaced by placebo injections (water in this case), a classically conditioned rise in blood sugar would result.[5] Instead, what the researchers found when they performed this particular experiment was that blood sugar actually decreased, which at first glance might appear to suggest that something besides a psychologically conditioned placebo effect was occurring.

Fortunately, the placebo effect was safe. The theory was correct, the prediction was wrong. Why? Because the repeated injections of glucose conditioned the body to respond as soon as possible to the set of external cues suggesting that the threat of high blood glucose levels was imminent (just as Pavlov's dogs salivated due to the promise of food, thus were getting their stomachs ready for the arrival of undigested food). Hence once this conditioning had occurred, the subsequent placebo injection alerted the central nervous system to begin the process of directing the body to secrete insulin and thereby to decrease blood sugar. Put another way, since the placebo contained no sugar, the released insulin had the effect of lowering the body's blood sugar. Hence the conditioned response (insulin) to this experimentally contrived and bogus threat was the exact response that should have occurred to this type of placebo effect.[6] So while most of the conditioned placebo effects we will be considering in this book aren't this complicated, it is worth remembering that they *can* be.

Immune Response in Mice

Few things seem further from our personal control or our imaginations than our immune system, but the truth is that even it can be conditioned. In a now famous series of experiments, a team of investigators fed water-deprived mice a harmless solution of saccharin-laced water followed by injections of a drug known to suppress the animals' immune system. This process was repeated for several days while another group of control mice were not subjected to this conditioning. Instead, the control mice were injected with a saline solution, which should have no effect upon the immune system.[7]

All of the mice (both those that were exposed to conditioning and those that were not) were then given the saccharin water and subsequently exposed to a toxic agent designed to generate an immune response in the form of released antibodies, which fight foreign substances that the body perceives to be potential threats to its functioning. The mice that had come to associate the saccharin drink with the immune-suppressing agent released significantly *fewer* antibodies than those that had not been conditioned. While certainly not conclusive proof of the existence of the placebo effect in human immunology, this series of experiments does suggest that more biological functions can be conditioned than previously suspected.

Direct Comparisons of the Effectiveness of Different Placebos

The placebo effect and drug effects are not mutually exclusive. It has often been speculated that even effective drugs possess placebo effects in addition to their specific biochemical reactions. It has also been assumed that certain therapies have greater placebo components than others. Bernard Finneson, in a classic text on surgery and pain, for example, described surgery as the possessing the strongest placebo effect in medicine, and there is some evidence that surgical placebos (e.g., the implantation of inactive pacemakers, irrelevant inner ear surgery as compared to the actual surgical insertion of drainage tubes, and sham artery-rerouting procedures in heart surgery) do indeed produce what appear to be extremely potent placebo effects.[8] It has also been suggested that CAM procedures and antidepressants (combined with the subjective nature of their outcomes) are close seconds to surgery, but at this point these are nothing more than unsubstantiated conjectures.[9]

In fact, the absence of no-treatment control groups in this research prevents us from knowing for sure that even the supposedly documented effects emanating from any of the research's placebo groups (surgical or otherwise) are actually placebo effects per se and not due to such artifacts as natural history.

There is one line of research, however, that directly compares one type of placebo with another. This is relevant to the question at hand because if there is a difference between two types of placebos, then that difference must be interpreted as evidence that there is such a thing as a placebo effect. What else could explain how one placebo could produce better outcomes than another when both are pharmacologically and physiologically inactive?

Based upon a comprehensive review of this research of this literature, there is at least some evidence (1) that administering a placebo more frequently will produce better outcomes than administering the same placebo less frequently, (2) that some pill colors induce greater placebo effects than others, (3) that placebos in capsule form are more effective than those constituted as pills, (4) that bigger placebo pills are more effective than smaller ones, and (5) that injected placebos produce stronger effects than orally ingested placebos.[10] The fact that most of these effects are based upon single, small-scale studies makes the validity of this line of research difficult to evaluate, however.

But recently there has been a large, high-quality trial funded by the National Center for Complementary and Alternative Medicine that directly contrasted two placebos—one involving the classic placebo pill and one involving an elaborate sham acupuncture procedure. Employing adults with arm pain due to repetitive use, the study found that pain symptoms improved more in the placebo acupuncture group than they did in the placebo pill group.[11] This finding was interpreted by the investigators as confirmation of the hypothesis that all placebos are not created equally, a conjecture that had been previously advanced by the study's lead investigator (i.e., that some procedural placebos such as surgery or acupuncture are more potent than simple placebo pills).[12] Unfortunately, since it wasn't possible to blind the practitioners administering the placebo acupuncture procedure (while presumably it was possible to blind the individuals passing out the placebo pills), this study may have actually documented the importance of double-blinding, the fact that some placebos are more potent than others, or both. Nevertheless, for our purposes, all of these potential explanations are supportive of the existence of a placebo effect—whether emanating from the practitioner or from the form of the placebo itself.

Desire or Motivation for Pain Relief

While related to expectations (which, as noted before, is a term that figures prominently in our definitions of what a placebo is in the first place), there is some evidence that people's desire (which can be conceptualized as motivation or perceived need) for pain relief also contributes to the magnitude of the placebo effect. The most direct evidence for this involved a laboratory experiment in which investigators manipulated both motivation and expectancy to observe their effects upon perceived pain relief resulting from the receipt of a placebo. Both factors appeared to contribute independently to the placebo response.[13]

There is also an intriguing genre of research suggesting that the desire or motivation to improve one's health may be an important factor in eliciting placebo effects. This supposition is related to those studies showing that patients who comply with their medical regimens (i.e., are conscientious in taking their medications) tend to improve more than patients who do not. This in itself isn't particularly surprising, since if a medication is worth anything, taking it regularly at prescribed doses *should* result in improvement. However, this relationship holds even for people who have been randomized to receive placebos—that is, patients who conscientiously take their placebo tablets tend to improve more than those who don't, even though there is absolutely no medical reason why this should happen.[14] Thus to me it seems safe to conclude that either desire and motivation for improvement *or*—and this is a huge *or*—beliefs in the efficacy of a prescribed treatment (which in turn affect compliance) play a role in eliciting the placebo effect.

Placebo Effects for Conditions Other than Pain

While there is no question that the evidence for both placebo and CAM therapeutic effects is considerably stronger for pain than for any other symptom, this by no means implies that there is *no* evidence for a placebo effect for other conditions. Personally, based upon experimental evidence, I would be shocked if there weren't a placebo effect in some of the drug treatments for depression and Parkinson's disease.[15] Moreover, some evidence exists (although it is based on findings that haven't been replicated) to show that placebos affect postoperative swelling, movement disorders, vital signs such as oral temperature and pulse, blood pressure, weight loss, exercise tolerance among heart patients, healing of ulcers, cholesterol reduction, blood sugar (as noted previously) and even the production of its negative symptoms such as headaches or drowsiness, decreased respiration, and cortisol levels commonly associated with the side effects of the drugs these placebos (which are now sometimes called nocebos) are designed to mimic.[16]

I have labeled as indirect evidence all of the results of the research discussed so far in this chapter because I am not convinced that there has been sufficient, carefully controlled research involving these individual conditions. I have included it only as a means of rounding out our discussion of the placebo effect, rather than presenting it as definitively demonstrating that there is indeed such a thing. To accomplish this task, let me briefly mention at least a few studies that, in my judgment, present the most scientifically defensible direct evidence addressing the existence of the placebo effect.

DIRECT EVIDENCE THAT THE PLACEBO EFFECT EXISTS

Physicians have long been taught that authoritative and/or positive presentation of a treatment regimen to a patient produces better therapeutic results than do neutral or equivocal messages. And unlike a lot of our other cherished assumptions, this one has a considerable number of experiments substantiating it. One of the earliest controlled studies of this sort occurred in the 1980s and involved comparing the effects of positive versus negative physician-patient interactions.

General Practice Consultations: Is There Any Point in Being Positive?

K. B. Thomas

In this study, patients with minor illnesses that would normally resolve themselves within a few days (e.g., colds or minor aches and pains) were randomly assigned to one of two groups when they arrived at their physician's office. Group 1 patients were all "given a firm diagnosis and told confidently that they would be better in a few days," while group 2 patients were all given a "negative consultation" in which the physician told the patients, "I cannot be certain just what is wrong with you."[17]

The results couldn't have been more straightforward: two weeks later, the patients who received the positive messages (group 1) reported having recovered significantly faster than those who got the negative or neutral message (group 2).[18] This basic effect has been validated several times in different ways with the same, somewhat less than earth-shattering conclusion: physicians are able to elicit a placebo effect through positive therapeutic interactions with their patients.

But the trouble with this line of research is that we are still left with a nagging question: can a placebo help patients who are suffering from serious pain resulting from a serious illnesses? My favorite study addressing this issue was performed on patients recovering from what I think everyone would consider is a treatment capable of inducing serious pain: thoracic surgery for lung cancer.

Response Expectancies in Placebo Analgesia and Their Clinical Relevance

Antonella Pollo, Martina Amanzio, Anna Arslanian, Caterina Casadio, Giuliano Maggi, and Fabrizio Benedetti

Following recovery from anesthesia, everyone in this study was given an additional analgesic, and then an IV containing nothing but a saline (placebo) solution was begun and continued for three days. The patients were then randomly assigned to one of three groups that were identical except for what they were told about their "useless" IV: group 1 was told nothing at all about what was in the IV or what it was for, group 2 was told that the IV might be either a real analgesic *or* a placebo, and group 3 was told that the placebo infusion was really a powerful painkiller. Patients in all three groups were then allowed to request anesthesia as needed and were given it when they so requested. (This allowance was ethically necessary, since these were real patients recovering from real surgery.)[19] Over the course of the next three days, group 3 (the patients who thought their IV contained a powerful painkiller) required 34 percent less analgesia than group 1 (the patients who weren't told anything about the IV) and 16 percent less than group 2 (the patients who were unsure whether their IV was a placebo or a real painkiller).[20] These results are charted in Figure 9.1.

The authors concluded that it was the differences in verbal instructions, which in turn resulted in differences in expectation or belief (a necessary condition for a placebo effect), that resulted in the need for

Figure 9.1. Placebo Analgesic Effects Based upon Three Different Sets of Instructions

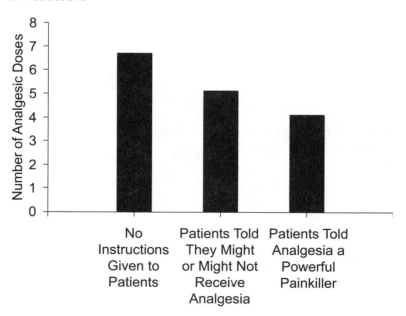

less pain medication. If there is an alternative explanation for these results, I haven't come up with it yet.

WHAT CAN WE CONCLUDE ABOUT THE RESEARCH PRESENTED IN THIS CHAPTER?

I'll let two people who've done a great deal more research on the placebo effect than I have answer this question. It is true that Donald Price and Henry Fields were alluding to a set of studies completely different from the ones I have just described.[21] However, their conclusion still rings true, which is that there are three primary factors involved in placebo analgesia:

> These include (1) classical conditioning effect that occurs without the subject's conscious awareness of the conditioned stimulus–unconditioned stimulus association; (2) a desire for a given treatment or agent to significantly relieve pain; and (3) the level of expectation that pain will be significantly relieved by such treatment or agent. Although we think that classical conditioning is a major determinant of the magnitude of the placebo effect, we propose that a combination of desire and expectation can be of equal if not greater importance.[22]

So, based upon the evidence that we've considered to this point, I believe we can accept as proven the first of four scientific principles that we will consider during the course of our quest:

> *Principle 1: The placebo effect is real and is capable of exerting at least a temporary pain reduction effect. It occurs only in the presence of the belief that an intervention (or therapy) is capable of exerting this effect. This belief can be instilled through classical conditioning, or simply by the suggestion of a respected individual that this intervention (or therapy) can reduce pain.*

But even if there is, without question, such a thing as a placebo effect for pain (and probably for many other symptoms as well), those annoying biologists in our midst would still question what the biochemical mechanism of this effect is. They simply can't help themselves, because raising such a question is what biologists do. Let me try, then, to address that question in the next chapter.

CHAPTER TEN

A Biochemical Explanation for the Placebo Effect

So far I have succeeded in proving the obvious: there is such a thing as a placebo effect. Unfortunately, the answers to some other questions are not quite as obvious. For example:

1. *Is there any evidence regarding what the underlying psychological mechanism is that triggers the placebo effect?* We already know that expectations play a role, but what psychological phenomenon can explain how a mere expectation can be strong enough to trigger something as dramatic as the placebo effects we've seen, say, in the thoracic surgery study? Pavlov's work has given us a powerful hint in this regard, but just because dogs are our best friends doesn't mean that we can accept their drooling as direct evidence for a placebo effect for pain relief in humans.

And then, regardless of how the placebo effect is triggered:

2. *Is the pain relief that occurs from this placebo-engendered expectation real or imagined?* This has important implications when we get around to explaining how CAM therapies result in pain relief. It also has important implications if we ever need to rely on Occam's razor because I doubt if William would award the placebo effect many points in its explanatory contest against the

effects of CAM therapies if all we can say about its analgesic action is that it's due to the patient's imagination.

And, finally, *if* the placebo effect is not a total figment of people's imagination:

3. *Is there any biochemical explanation for any nonimaginary component of the placebo effect?* This is ultimately the most important question of all because it addresses the plausibility of the research presented in the last chapter.

THE PSYCHOLOGICAL MECHANISM UNDERLYING THE PLACEBO EFFECT

I've hinted at the importance of classical conditioning in engendering the placebo effect, referring to both Pavlov's original work and subsequent research involving the drug conditioning literature. Now it's time to discuss some research that *directly* implicates conditioning as the phenomenon's triggering mechanism, beginning with what I consider a definitive experiment in this regard.

An Analysis of Factors That Contribute to the Magnitude of Placebo Analgesia in an Experimental Paradigm

Donald Price, Irving Kirsch, Ann Duff, Guy Montgomery, and Sarah Nicholls

This experiment was published in the journal *Pain* in 1999.[1] The first author, Donald Price, is a recognized pain expert and has published some very insightful technical books on the subject.[2] More important for us here, he has produced some of the best research yet conducted regarding both the physiological and psychological mechanisms involved in the placebo effect. Despite this achievement, he once remarked to me that practically no one outside his immediate family has any idea of why he does what he does (which secretly made me quite jealous, since no one in my family even knows what I do, much less my motivations for doing it).

In any case, this study involved an extremely sophisticated laboratory inducement of experimental pain, using a thermal device that could administer an uncomfortable but transitory amount of pain tailored to the individual's pain tolerance. (All of which is a politically correct way of saying that the participants were burned, but not enough to leave a mark or for the pain to persist after the study was over.)

Recognizing that everyone reading this book won't share my passion for experimental design, I will report only those parts of the study that I consider essential to showing that a placebo effect can be classically conditioned.

The participants (college students) were told (by the experimenter, appropriately dressed in a white lab coat) that the study for which they had just volunteered was designed to evaluate "a new, topical, local anesthetic...for its pain-reducing effects." They were told the drug's name was Trivaricaine and that it had been "proven effective in pre-liminary studies at other universities." Of course, the "drug" was really a placebo that, in the authors' words, "was a mixture of iodine, oil of thyme, and water that produced a brownish, medicinal smelling effect when applied topically. This placebo concoction was placed in two medicine bottles labeled, 'Trivaricaine-A' and 'Trivaricaine-B: Approved for research purposes only.'" A third bottle contained only water and was creatively labeled C.

After they were familiarized with the equipment and the pain in-tensities to be used, participants were assessed for their pain thresholds and then the experiment began. Three areas on the participants' fore-arms were marked via labels on Band-Aids, although the locations of these areas were rotated randomly from person to person. Then the trickery really began: the investigators informed the participants "that bottle C was a control wetting solution [which certainly adequately de-scribes water] and that bottles A and B contained different strengths of the local analgesic 'Trivaricaine.'" So in effect, what we have is three experimental "treatments" consisting of a strong placebo (strong only because the participants were told that it was a strong analgesic), a weak placebo, and no placebo (or no treatment).

Unlike the other experiments we've discussed so far, however, here all the study participants received all three treatments. In other words, everyone was administered the pain suggested by the "medication's" description. Thus, the "strong analgesia" location on each person's arm received the mildest (least painful) temperature setting, the "weak analgesia" location received a considerably more uncomfortable setting, and the final location (at which point patients were told that were they receiving no pain medication at all, only the "wetting solution") received the most intensive, painful stimulus of all.

What was Price doing here? He was creating a placebo effect by *reinforcing* what he had told the patients *would* happen. None of the medications had any pain-relieving capabilities at all, but the participants didn't know that. When he told his participants that they were receiving a strong medication, he burned them less than when he told them they were receiving a weak medication. When he told them they were receiving no medication at all, he burned the hell out of them. So the patients experienced exactly what they expected to experience based upon what they were told to expect. And the pain "relief" they experienced wasn't in their imaginations; it was very, very real. Of course, the pain "relief" they were experiencing was provided by Price's devious manipulation of his thermal machine, not by the fake medications. But how could his participants know that?

So what we have here is a classical conditioning experience, very similar to Pavlov's dogs except that instead of getting food, Price's participants got uncomfortable "thermal stimuli." Then, once our experimenter could be sure that his participants believed in the effectiveness of his fake (placebo) medications and would expect considerable pain relief from the strong placebo, the stage was set to find out if these expectations themselves could actually influence the amount of pain experienced.

To do this, Price told his participants that they would receive some additional heat applications to each area treated by one of the three "medications." So naturally, everyone knew exactly what to expect because they had already experienced these "medication" effects. This time around, however, Price administered exactly the same amount of pain at each medication site; the amount of real pain relief due to the medications that could be expected from these sites was the same too, which was *zero*. What happened? The results, using the standard ten-point visual analog scale (shown previously, in Figure 3.2) used in hospitals, drug research, and CAM research, are presented in Table 10.1 for both the conditioning phase (the second column, where you'd *expect* there to be a lot of difference in the amount of pain experienced because participants really were administered different amounts of pain) and the placebo phase (the third column, where you wouldn't expect to see any difference in pain—at least if you didn't suspect there was such

Table 10.1. Experimentally Induced Pain Intensity for Three Placebo Groups

Treatment Groups*	Rated Pain Intensity, Conditioning Phase**	Rated Pain Intensity, Placebo or Postconditioning Phase***
No placebo	6.2	4.6
Weak placebo	4.5	4.0
Strong placebo	2.5	3.3

 * *Each participant received all three treatments.*

 ** *Actual pain varied between groups. Higher numbers indicate more perceived pain.*

*** *Actual pain was the same for each group. Higher numbers indicate more perceived pain.*

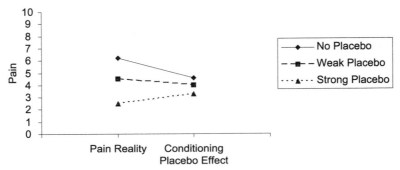

Figure 10.1. Weak versus Strong Placebo Effect for Pain

a thing as a placebo effect operating—because there really *weren't* any differences in the amount of pain administered).

Or see Figure 10.1, for those of you who are more graphically oriented.

As expected, there were major differences in the amount of pain experienced in the conditioning phase. Why? Because there were major differences in the amount of pain administered. The truly interesting finding involves the significant differences in the amount of pain the participants experienced in the placebo or postconditioning phase. Why? Again, because there were absolutely no differences in the amount of pain (or heat) administered in this phase of the experiment.

How did the investigators explain these results occurring during the placebo phase of the trial? Since the experiment had been so carefully designed, there was only one plausible explanation: the pain differences the second time around were due exclusively to the participants' expectations that there would be a difference in the amount of pain experienced. This perfectly fits our preferred definition of the placebo effect, which again is: "a pharmacologically [or physiologically] inactive substance that can have a therapeutic effect if administered to a patient who believes that he or she is receiving an effective treatment."[3] The inactive substance in this case was the placebo called Trivaricaine. And we know that the participants believed that they were receiving an effective treatment because of the elaborate hoax constructed by Price and his colleagues.

I personally can't think of any reason other than the existence of a placebo effect that could explain why these differences should exist in the placebo phase of the experiment. (Take my word for it as a bio-statistician: the differences are real and would occur by chance alone less than one time out of several thousand experiments.) I also find it quite impressive that these placebo-phase results (in column 3 of Table 10.1) closely mirror the results due to the actual pain experienced in the conditioning phase (column 2), and also that the placebo differences observed (column 3) are slightly less than the actual levels found in column 2. (Remember the drug conditioning studies mentioned in the last chapter? The results of those studies showed that the placebo effects mirrored the real drug effects but were always smaller in magnitude.)

So how does all of this apply to placebo effects occurring in clinical settings where physicians (or CAM practitioners) don't cause pain but instead attempt to reduce it? First, the results of the Price study suggest why doctors are so good at eliciting placebo effects. We have all been conditioned to expect our physicians to help us based upon the fact that they really have helped us in the past. (Or at least we think they did, based upon natural history and the other inferential artifacts discussed earlier.) We have, in other words, been conditioned, à la Pavlov's dogs, to expect the medications they give us to work. Second, these findings explain how CAM therapists (even if they were administering nothing more potent than a New Age version of this study's "medication C") could inadvertently trick their patients into believing that their pain has been relieved. And then, based upon their patients' response, these very real placebo effects represented by column 3 could reinforce the CAM therapists' belief in the effectiveness of their therapies. Such therapies may be engendering nothing more than the expectation that they will reduce pain by elaborate explanations, promises, and ceremonies.

But there is yet another finding in Price's study that may have even more applicability to CAM. This involves a quirk in how we remember

Table 10.2. A Comparison of the Remembrance of the Placebo Effect with the Actual Experience

Groups	Conditioning Phase	Postconditioning Phase	Memories of Postconditioning Phase
No placebo	6.2	4.6	6.8
Weak placebo	4.5	4.0	4.7
Strong placebo	2.5	3.3	3.0

our pain experiences and hence the relief that we think we experience from things such as CAM therapies. Price and his associates added one small wrinkle to their trial. Exactly two minutes following the post-conditioning placebo phase, they asked the study participants to try to recall how much pain they had suffered a couple of minutes before, in the second (or placebo) phase of the study. These results are presented in Table 10.2, which is nothing more than Table 10.1 with a fourth column added to represent the participants' memories of the placebo phase. I've also added Figure 10.2 for those readers who find graphs easier to interpret than tables full of numbers.

Figure 10.2. Actual Placebo Effect versus Memory of Placebo Effect

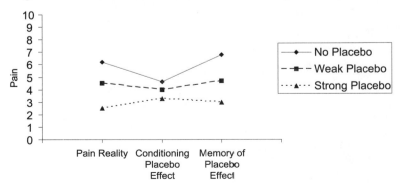

Admittedly, I'm a bit on the strange side, but I get excited every time I see what happens to the solid line (no placebo) between the second point (the placebo phase, which reflects the success of classical conditioning) and the third point (where participants had to rely upon their memories of what occurred just two minutes earlier). Why?

> *The remembrance of the pain suffered at what the participants thought was the no-treatment point (of course, no one in the study at any time actually got any real treatment) was greater than they actually experienced.*

Then I get even more excited when I look at the memory of the pain experienced, as witnessed by the dotted line (the strong placebo group), which may be used to reflect a CAM treatment experience. Here the memory of the pain that the participants reported experiencing following what they thought was a treatment was actually less than they experienced. They basically remembered the no-placebo (or "no-treatment") pain as greater than it really was, and they remembered the pain at the strong-placebo (CAM) point as less than it really was. Viewed from another perspective, the strongest placebo effect observed in this study (strong placebo versus no placebo) occurred when participants relied on their memories of what they experienced ($6.8 - 3.0 = 3.8$) compared to when they actually experienced it ($4.6 - 3.3 = 1.3$).

And as illustrated in Figures 10.1 and 10.2 (and similar to the earlier research dealing with the conditioning of drug effects), the differences due to the conditioned placebo effect (the second set of points) are considerably less than the differences in actual pain suffered during the first phase (the first set of points). The important finding for us here, however, is:

> *The memory of the pain relief afforded by the placebo "treatments" was considerably more dramatic than the pain relief the participants actually experienced at the time. This means that if CAM therapies really are placebos, their recipients will remember them as being more effective than they actually were.*

I should mention that this effect for the remembrance of pain and of its relief is not unique to this study but has been independently documented by other investigators as well.[4]

IS THE PAIN RELIEF ELICITED BY THE PLACEBO EFFECT REAL OR IMAGINARY?

As impressive as these results are, they leave a huge gap in our understanding regarding *how* the placebo effect manifests itself once it has been triggered. All of which leads us back to the final two questions posed at the beginning of this chapter:

Is the placebo effect real or imaginary?

And:

If it is real, what happens inside the body that actually results in pain relief?

One perfectly reasonable response to either question might be: "Who cares?" We know that a placebo effect occurs. We know that it occurs in the presence of an expectation of therapeutic benefit. We know that these expectations can be conditioned. Who cares if patients only imagine the pain relief effects that are attributable to placebos? Or if the effects are real, who cares what in the body makes them occur?

We have to care because we are in the process of weighing the plausibility and credibility of imperfect evidence impacting the question of whether any CAM therapies are more effective than a placebo. There is already plenty of evidence to demonstrate what the psychological mechanism most likely is for the placebo and to explain that this same psychological mechanism *could* account for the presumed effects of CAM therapies. For a hard-nosed neurobiological researcher, however, psychological explanations such as classically conditioned expectations of pain relief that somehow become self-fulfilling prophecies really don't count for very much. To say that the placebo effect is generated by expectations doesn't identify a biomedical mechanism of action either. A biologist (or a scientifically oriented physician, for that matter) would repeat the same question: what caused the pain relief?

Of course, we could impatiently answer, "The mind does it, dummy!" But the next question out of the annoying biologist's mouth will inevitably be: "*How* does the mind do it?" We could argue that the benefits that people attribute to both CAM and placebos are largely imaginary, a function of flawed memories, or both. We could even take the CAM route of positing some as yet unmeasured energy coursing through the universe (or through an entire physiological system within the body that has somehow escaped detection up to this point) to explain the relief of pain. Or we could argue that it is enough that we've demonstrated that the placebo effect exists and that is indistinguishable from CAM therapeutic effects, and that questions about the underlying biochemical causes of those effects aren't especially relevant to the real experience of pain relief.

The fact is that there are some very serious scientists walking among us who don't believe that anything is real that isn't regulated by a protein of some sort. Fortunately for us, some of them have studied the placebo effect and its biochemical mechanisms, so I will discuss their research before moving on to the evidence addressing whether or not there is such a thing as a CAM therapeutic effect over and above those that are attributable to the placebo effect.

THE POPPY FIELDS OF THE MIND

Often in basic scientific research (which sometimes appears to have no applicability to anything except knowledge for knowledge's sake), arriving at an answer to one question can help resolve other questions that the research was not intended to address. In understanding the placebo effect, for example, we get some unexpected help from work done without any thought to placebos. Physiologists have known for some time of the existence of a number of defensive chemical substances (e.g., endorphins, catecholamines, cortisol, adrenaline) that the body has at its disposal to dampen the potentially deleterious effects of pain. They also know from where these substances are released, which is generally along what is called the hypothalamic-pituitary-adrenal axis. They know some of the environmental triggers that activate this axis (pain, fear of a perceived threat, or other strong emotion), and they know the chemistry of what happens following this activation. So a natural place to look for any analgesic effects that are not introduced by an outside source (such as an injected or ingested drug) would appear to be among this biochemical cadre.

The search actually began during the late 1970s and early 1980s when a number of investigators were able to demonstrate that a drug called naloxone could at least partially block the placebo effect.[5] This is relevant because naloxone is an opioid antagonist, which means that it is capable of nullifying the analgesic effects of opioid-based drugs such as morphine (naloxone is still sometimes used to treat heroin overdoses) as well as of the substances produced by the body's very own opioid system, which itself had been discovered only a few years earlier.[6]

Let's add this arcane piece of knowledge to what we now know about the placebo effect, which is that it exists and that it can be triggered by our expectations of therapeutic benefit, and let's surmise that what is triggered (at least with respect to pain relief) may involve the body's opioid system. Then let's look at the recent research of another group of investigators who (based upon the pioneering work just mentioned) devised a most eloquent experiment to address all three of these points at the same time. This experiment did something else equally important—it demonstrated that the analgesic effects resulting from placebos were real, not imaginary. At the risk of repetitiveness, let's recall that none of the research we've discussed in any detail up to this point dispels the possibility that the entire placebo effect could be a purely psychological phenomenon. In other words, in humans at least, conditioning and suggestion may cause people to believe that they are experiencing less pain while, in reality, their nervous systems are processing pain stimuli just as intense as those experienced by people who haven't been tricked into believing that they are receiving a real analgesic therapy. (Of course, we would be hard pressed to explain some of the indirect evidence from the last chapter, such as the immune responses to placebos observed, but this research is outside our primary purview at this point.)

Here, then, is the experiment (backed by the early research mentioned above)[7] that I submit as the benchmark with which to compare later the physiological mechanisms proposed to explain any non-placebo-initiated analgesic effects of CAM therapies.

Response Variability to Analgesics: A Role for Non-Specific Activation of Endogenous Opioids

Martina Amanzio, Antonella Pollo, Giuliano Maggi, and Fabrizio Benedetti

This experiment was designed to see if the placebo effect could be chemically blocked under carefully controlled conditions.[8] Its underlying premise is that something has to be real before it can be chemically blocked, it has to be triggered before we know it is real, and so therefore it is a good guess that the thing being chemically blocked is the "something" that was triggered in the first place. Like Donald Price before them, these investigators got around the ethical considerations of causing pain in patients in desperate need of pain relief by recruiting healthy volunteers who were willing to allow pain to be experimentally induced in them (or, more accurately, were willing to induce it in themselves).

Then, prior to the beginning of the experiment, the researchers inserted an IV line through which drugs could be run. Once this was done, the investigators began their experiment by placing a blood pressure cuff on each of the volunteers and connecting it to a hand-squeezable bulb. Each squeeze consequently increased the cuff pressure by a standardized amount—hence the participants had a mechanism by which they could induce a precisely measurable amount of pressure until they judged the resulting pain to have become intolerable. Since they were instructed to squeeze the bulb once every four seconds until this masochistic point was reached, the elapsed time between the first and last squeezes yielded an extremely precise indication of pain tolerance.

Following an initial dry run to ascertain each individual's pain tolerance, the participants were randomly assigned to one of the six groups discussed below. If you're not willing to take the results on faith, you'll probably have to read the following sections a couple of times. Certainly I did when I first ran into this particular experiment.

Group 1: no-treatment control. Here, nothing was done to the participants except have them repeat the dry run to obtain a second measure of pain tolerance. The purpose of this group was to provide a basis for comparison for the other groups regarding what would happen in the *absence* of any pain medication or any placebo effect. (This group was necessary because all of the other experimental groups would also be measured twice, once before the treatment and once afterward. It would not be reasonable, for example, to use a zero change in pain tolerance as the basis for comparing the remainder of the treatment groups since the simple act of measuring people twice might produce different results the second time around.)

Group 2: hidden naloxone (opioid blocker) only. The purpose of this group was to assess whether or not the opioid-blocking drug had any effect upon pain in and of itself. This was important to assess because naloxone might be expected to actually *increase* pain by blocking the body's opioid system. As you've probably guessed, the researchers are eventually going to attempt to block the placebo effect using naloxone and thereby increase the participants' pain. The inclusion of the naloxone-only group is therefore necessary to ensure that this increased pain is not due to naloxone itself rather than to the blocked placebo effect. (The administration of naloxone had to be hidden—which means that it was run through the participants' IV lines unannounced—

because to announce that something was coming through the line might induce a placebo effect in and of itself. Theoretically, this group should witness the same change, or lack thereof, in pain tolerance as the no-treatment control, group 1.)

Group 3: hidden non-opioid analgesic. The individuals in this group received through their IVs an effective analgesic (called ketorolac) that was not opioid-based. The participants were not informed that this was happening. (Obviously this group should manifest some very real increased pain tolerance simply because ketorolac is a scientifically proven, effective analgesic. It was necessary to include this group because the investigators needed to measure how effective this drug was in the absence of a placebo effect. Why? Because they were going to define the placebo effect in terms of how much the expectation of relief could add to the drug's effectiveness, which is why the participants in this group were not told that they were receiving the drug.)

Group 4: hidden non-opioid analgesic plus hidden opioid blocker. The participants in this group received ketorolac (as in group 3) followed by naloxone (which they also weren't aware they were receiving). (Note: At first glance this group may seem redundant with the last one, but the investigators needed to demonstrate that indeed the opioid blocker did not affect the non-opioid analgesic's pain reduction effects. It was necessary to demonstrate this anyway since William of Occam has counseled us against making unnecessary assumptions, which in research such as this translates to employing controls that prevent us from taking anything for granted. The researchers expected the subjects in this group to experience the same increases in pain tolerance as those in group 3, since both were getting a real analgesic, although unannounced. Both should, however, obviously display a greater pain tolerance than groups 1 and 2.)

Group 5: announced administration of the non-opioid analgesic, no opioid blocker. Reflecting the procedure used for postsurgical patients in the experiment discussed in the last chapter,[9] the participants were told that they were about to receive an effective analgesic *before* they began another round of self-inflicted pain. (As you may have guessed, this was the primary group needed to demonstrate the existence of a placebo effect. Even though virtually the same investigators had already demonstrated that this procedure elicited a placebo effect in the post-surgical study, it was absolutely necessary to reestablish this fact here; again, nothing can be taken on faith in experiments such as these. Also, just because this effect manifests itself in a clinical situation—that is, with real physicians and real patients—does not mean that it will do so in an artificial, experimental one. In any event, our Italian friends hypothesized that this group would exceed all of the others with respect to pain tolerance because it involved both the use of an effective analgesic *and* the placebo effect. Its members, therefore, *should* be able to tolerate more pain than both group 3, which received unannounced administration of the non-opioid analgesic, and group 4, which received unannounced administration of the non-opioid analgesic followed by an irrelevant opioid blocker—remembering that there should be no difference between groups 3 and 4. Of course, group 5's members should exhibit more pain tolerance than groups 1 and 2 as well.)

Group 6: announced administration of the non-opioid analgesic plus hidden administration of the opioid blocker. This group constituted the crux of the entire experiment. Participants were told that they were receiving an effective analgesic but not that it would be accompanied by an opioid (placebo) blocker. (Note: This was important because this group's pain tolerance should be less than that of the participants assigned to group 5, even though both groups received an effective analgesic accompanied by the inducement of expected benefits therefrom. Group 5 should have the benefit of both analgesia derived from the drug and analgesia derived from the placebo effect, because participants were told that they were getting an effective painkiller. Group 6, however, should receive the benefit from the drug only if—and this is a very big *if*—the placebo's analgesic effect was opioid in nature, in which case the hidden administration of naloxone should block the placebo effect even though the psychological condition that triggers it—the expectation of benefit—is present. Group 6 should therefore be no different from group 4 (hidden non-opioid analgesic plus opioid blocker) because the two groups were conceptually the same: both should receive analgesia from the drug but not from the placebo. Why? Because participants in group 4 weren't told they were getting the drug (and hence couldn't have a placebo effect) and people in group 6 couldn't have a placebo effect because it would be chemically blocked if the placebo effect's pain reduction mechanism was opioid in nature. The same would hold true for the comparison between group 6 and group 3: group 3 got the drug but not the placebo because these participants weren't told that they were getting the drug. Remember, naloxone is completely irrelevant to all of these groups except group 6 because it should have no effect upon the analgesic drug used in this study.)

By now you probably desperately wish that you had chosen either science or statistics as a profession. If you'll bear with me for just a page or two longer, however, I'll make you even more jealous. First, let's summarize the researchers' prediction with respect to pain tolerance: pain tolerance in group 5 (which received drug plus placebo pain relief) should be *greater* than in groups 3, 4, and 6 (all of which received an analgesic drug but no placebo), and it should be greater in groups 3 through 6 than in groups 1 and 2 (neither of which received any pain relief at all).

Incredibly, as depicted in Table 10.3 (and Figure 10.3), this is exactly the result that was obtained: pain tolerance (which in this case is comparable to pain relief) was greatest when the participants had access to both the drug and the unblocked placebo effect (group 5). Next, pain tolerance (or pain relief) was greater for participants who received an effective drug but had their placebo effect blocked (groups 3, 4, and 6) than it was for the poor souls (groups 1 and 2) receiving no pain relief at all.

I should repeat the fact at this point that in research, means of entire groups containing different people are never identical to each other, even if the drugs or interventions to which they are exposed are identical. For this reason, investigators need biostatisticians such as your

Table 10.3. Pain Tolerance Due to Drug Alone (Groups 3, 4, 6) Versus Drug Plus Placebo (Group 5) Versus No Drug or Placebo (Groups 1, 2)

Groups	Pain Tolerance*
1. No treatment (control)	12.0 minutes
2. No analgesic, but hidden opioid blocker	11.8 minutes
3. Hidden analgesic, no opioid blocker	17.0 minutes
4. Hidden analgesic, hidden opioid blocker	17.2 minutes
5. Announced analgesic, no opioid blocker	20.4 minutes
6. Announced analgesic, opioid blocker	17.3 minutes

These values are only approximate since they were estimated from a graph.

author to subject their results to statistical analysis (performed by computers) to determine whether or not the obtained differences are due to chance. It is at this point that the results of an experiment are blessed as statistically significant or cursed as not significant by people in my profession.

In this case, the difference between groups 1 and 2 was judged by the computer to be so small that it should not be considered as significant. The same was true for the differences between groups 3, 4, and 6. Group 5 differed significantly from all of the other groups, however, and groups 3, 4, and 6 differed significantly from groups 1 and 2.

So what is the interpretation here? First, there is a placebo effect that can be triggered by telling people that they are getting an effective analgesic, but of course we already knew that from comparing group 5 and group 3, not to mention the research presented in the last chapter. Second, at least part of the physiological basis for the placebo effect is opioid in nature (group 5 versus group 6), although most pain experts already knew this because of the pioneering placebo work done over the past two and a half decades.[10] Nowhere in the annals of science,

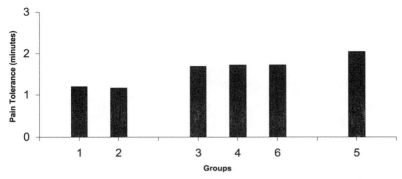

Figure 10.3. Illustration of a Possible Biochemical Explanation for the Placebo Effect

however, has this entire package ever been so eloquently demonstrated as in the study by Amanzio and colleagues.

Thus, since we know that no opioids were introduced into the body during this relatively brief laboratory experiment, we now have a biochemical mechanism to explain how the placebo effect is able to manifest itself. That mechanism is none other than the body's own poppy field—that is, its ability to produce opioids.

Some Limitations of This Experiment

As impressive as this work is, it does not categorically prove beyond the shadow of any doubt that the body's release of opioids is the mechanism of action for the placebo effect. There could be other mechanisms as well. It does not even categorically prove that the endogenous (naturally occurring) opioid system is one of the mechanisms of action for the placebo effect since our experimenters did not actually observe (or measure) the naloxone suppressing the endogenous opioids. Perhaps the naloxone was blocking something completely different, something that we don't even suspect or know about and hence can't get at through the process of elimination. Perhaps there is a mysterious, as yet unmeasured source of energy in the universe that the naloxone blocked. Perhaps it was those damn aliens who, unbeknownst to anyone, landed in Milan and abducted the entire research team and their experimental participants. But how would you personally feel about championing one or more of these alternative explanations in the presence of our stern fourteenth-century monk? Fortunately, another, even more recent line of research prevents us from facing this embarrassing possibility.

Brain Scans Documenting Endogenous Opioids as a Placebo Mechanism

There is a fascinating, rapidly progressing line of work addressing what goes on in the brain when we are introduced to a placebo. I will not discuss these studies in great detail because I consider them more supportive of the work just discussed than definitive in their own right and because, in my opinion (and probably my opinion only), research involving brain scans does not yet involve an exact science.

The first of these studies of which I am aware was published in *Science* in 2002 and employed positron emission tomography (PET) scans of nine patients in order to determine whether increased activity could be observed in specific areas of the brain after both an opioid-based analgesic medication and a behaviorally induced placebo effect were administered in the presence of experimentally induced pain.[11] The investigators were successful in pinpointing the location of increased activity following the introduction of a successful placebo (that is, one that resulted in pain relief), primarily in and around an area of the brain called the rotral anterior cingulated cortex—known for some time to contain a high concentration of opioid receptors.

Two years later a pair of functional magnetic resonance imaging (fMRI) studies took a slightly different tack with somewhat larger samples (twenty-four and thirty-two participants, respectively) and demonstrated that decreased brain activity in pain-sensitive brain regions could be observed in the presence of successful placebo analgesia.[12]

Then, the very next year (2005), a team of investigators reported the first *direct* evidence, using PET scans and molecular imaging, that the placebo effect is at least partially explained by the brain's endogenous opioid system.[13] In a nutshell, what these investigators did was inject participants with a substance capable of chemically signaling when the opioid-releasing structures in the brain do indeed release their opioids and also of being traced via a PET scan. They employed this strategy three times: (1) at baseline, when nothing was happening; (2) following the introduction of painful infusions of saltwater into healthy volunteers for up to an hour; and (3) following another long pain stimulus accompanied by the bogus expectation of pain relief (i.e., a placebo).

Two things happened: the participants reported experiencing a significantly lower level of pain during the placebo session, and a significantly greater activation of specific opioid-releasing structures was documented during the placebo session than during the session in which no expectation of pain relief was present. Thus, while not as intricate as the six-group naloxone study reported in the last section, this study did not have to "back into" the conclusion that body's endogenous opioid system was one factor in placebo analgesia; the researchers observed it (more or less) directly.

And the evidence keeps accumulating. In 2006 a study reminiscent of one of Price's sophisticated designs administered the now familiar "noxious thermal stimuli" in an elaborate sequence of intensities and locations to provide baseline information on optimal experimental temperatures and to ensure that participants could reliably differentiate among these temperatures. They were then treated with sham acupuncture accompanied by assurances of the effectiveness of that therapy for reducing pain. They were also told (for experimental purposes) that acupuncture would work only on the side of the arm in which the needles were inserted (remember that these were sham needles). Then, borrowing a page from Price's playbook, they "surreptitiously decreased the temperature of all noxious stimuli by 4–6°C on whichever side of the arm had received treatment [placebo side] but used the same stimuli temperature as before on the non-treated side [control side]." This, of course, was done to trick patients into believing that the placebo was really decreasing their pain. (No real acupuncture was administered in this study, only placebo acupuncture.)

Finally, the deceptive part of the experiment was repeated while the participants were actually in the fMRI scanner so that the investigators could determine what was going on in the brain when this intricately conceived placebo effect was taking place. The investigators found that indeed there were statistically significant reductions in participants' self-reported pain as a result of their placebo procedures, and also that this placebo-induced reduction in pain was associated with increased activity in an area of the brain known to "contain a high level of opioid receptors," leading the authors to conclude that their "results support the view that endogenous opioids may be involved in expectancy enhanced acupuncture placebo analgesia.'[14]

WHERE WE ARE NOW

What we now have is high-quality, independently validated evidence supporting the hypotheses that there is such a thing as a placebo effect and that at least one of the analgesic mechanisms of action for the placebo effect is the body's own opioid system. I include the qualifier "at least one" not simply to hedge my bets or to avoid criticism but because no one of whom I am aware—certainly not Donald Price nor our Italian colleagues—claims that that this mechanism is the *only* factor in placebo analgesia. That we have one such explanation that any competent neurophysiologist would judge to be plausible, based upon evidence that any reputable scientist would judge to be quite credible, however, gives us our second crucial scientific principle:

Principle 2: The placebo effect has a plausible, biochemical mechanism of action (at least for pain reduction), and that mechanism of action is the body's endogenous opioid system.

So now the task before us is to determine if the scientific literature produces comparably definitive principles demonstrating the existence of CAM therapeutic effects and their biochemical mechanisms of action. Regardless of the answer, our story will then be at its end.

CHAPTER ELEVEN

What High-Quality Trials Reveal About CAM

We are now ready to examine the evidence regarding whether CAM therapies are capable of producing health benefits over and above those that can be attributed to the placebo effect. This is a much more daunting task than it appears on the surface because of the number of clinical trials that have been conducted and the difficulties involved in sorting out the CAM studies. As of the end of 2002, for example, there were more than 350,000 published trials in one research registry alone, with several thousand more being added each year.[1]

But the sheer amount of research isn't the real root of the problem. The true difficulty of making sense of CAM research involves the conflicting research produced by *bias*.

BIAS

Some types of bias are obvious. Whenever people study something that can be sold for a profit, there is a very real possibility of bias creeping into their research. Thus it probably won't shock anyone to learn that drug research paid for by pharmaceutical companies produces more positive results—that is, greater benefits and fewer side effects—than does drug research paid for by public funds.[2] Nor would anyone be too surprised to learn that research conducted by advocates of a therapy tends to produce more positive results than trials conducted by more disinterested parties.

Sometimes research bias can be quite subtle and involve nothing more than putting a positive spin upon one's findings. Then again, sometimes it is incredibly blatant, involving the actual fabrication of data and even entire experiments. While the history of science is replete with examples of both, scientists in general are very poor at detecting blatant fraud in research and ultimately must rely upon independent replication to weed this problem out.[3] Unfortunately, we don't have the resources to do this routinely except for findings of earth-shattering proportions such as a major breakthrough in the treatment (or biochemical mechanism) of an incurable disease.

On the bright side, most scientists believe that downright fraud is relatively rare. Spinning one's results just beyond the limits of credibility, on the other hand, is disconcertingly common. And to be fair, there is no evidence to indicate that either practice is more endemic to CAM than to conventional medical research.

There are other sources of bias, however, that involve neither data fabrications nor positive spins. These, too, conspire to produce false positive results—which means that within the welter of published research there is a disproportionate percentage of positive findings breathlessly reporting that this or that CAM (or conventional) therapy is the greatest thing since sliced bread. So before we get down to examining the evidence, let's confront three of these unexpected sources of bias.

Bias from Scientific Acculturation (or the Lack Thereof)

Although seldom openly discussed outside scientific circles, one source of bias is cultural in nature, as witnessed by the fact that some countries and even whole continents tend to produce almost nothing but positive results. This has extremely serious implications for our present task because a significant amount of CAM research comes from these regions of the world—which means that we begin our search by encountering a built-in positive bias favoring CAM therapies.

While this statement may sound like a severe case of chauvinistic nationalism on your author's part, it is not a matter of opinion. In a 1998 article aptly titled "Do Certain Countries Produce Only Positive Results? A Systematic Review of Controlled Trials," Andrew Vickers (who at the time was working for the Research Council for Complementary Medicine in London) and his colleagues set out to ascertain if the nationality of the principal authors influenced the results of the trials they undertook.[4] They reviewed 252 published accounts of acupuncture trials, and the results of their survey appear in Table 11.1.

What I think these results demonstrate very definitively is that CAM investigators' countries of origin must be considered in the interpretation of CAM effectiveness trials. Chinese-speaking countries, for example, simply did not produce anything but positive acupuncture trials, while parts of Europe did not lag that far behind. And when Vickers and his colleagues repeated the analyses with a much larger sample of trials involving treatments other than acupuncture (most of which involved conventional medical treatments), they basically came up with the same results: 98 percent of conventional Chinese trials produced positive results, as did 97 percent of Russian trials.

So there is obviously something very strange going on here. Perhaps the investigators behind these studies never had the opportunity to receive a proper scientific education and especially to be acculturated into the scientific ethic via exposure to a principled, experienced mentor.[5] It should be noted that most of the studies Vickers referred to were conducted prior to the Consolidated Standards of Reporting Trials (CONSORT) statement, which laid out the best consensus among methodologists and statisticians about what constitutes high-quality RCT practice. These scientific procedures for conducting randomized, controlled trials are, one hopes, available to all scientists now.

Because this is a genuine problem in reviewing the evidence surrounding our CAM-versus-placebo question, I personally would have preferred to look at only CAM trials conducted by English-speaking and

Table 11.1. Positive CAM Results by Country/Region of Origin

Investigator's Origin	Number of Acupuncture Trials	Percentage of Positive Results
Non-U.S./non-U.K. English-speaking countries (Canada, Australia, New Zealand)	20	30%
United States	47	53%
Scandinavia (Sweden, Denmark, Finland)	47	55%
United Kingdom	20	60%
Other European countries (e.g., Russia, France, Germany)	62	78%
Asia (China, Hong Kong, Taiwan, Japan, Sri Lanka,* Vietnam)	52	98%
Other countries (Brazil, Israel, Nigeria)	3	100%

* Sri Lanka produced the only Asian CAM trial that was not positive.

Scandinavian investigators, which would have cut down the amount of evidence that needs to be considered by more than half. I compromised, however, and made the decision to limit the trials considered in this chapter to only those published in the most selective English-language research journals, in part because English is the language of science and in part because these journals do subscribe to the CONSORT statement and attempt to be quite selective with respect to the methodological quality of the articles they publish. That said, the next chapter considers worldwide evidence irrespective of country of origin.

And my reason for reviewing only selective journals? We have known for a long time that lower-quality clinical trials produce biased results and that the direction of that bias is—you guessed it—toward false positive results.[6] Thus journals that are more selective with respect to the quality of the trials they publish help to decrease bias and to safe-guard the validity of the results we need to consider.

Publication Bias

There is another source of bias that is probably responsible for contrib-uting more false positive results to a body of evidence than any other in existence, yet it has nothing to do with the conduct of research, the re-searcher's country of origin, or the subject matter involved. Instead, it deals exclusively with the publication process and the scientific reward system. It is of crucial importance for a task such as ours, which involves attempting to evaluate a large body of published research for the express purpose of coming up with a bottom-line conclusion about CAM effectiveness.

This miscreant is called publication bias, and it refers to a well-documented tendency for research journals to favor positive results (e.g., acupuncture helps arthritis sufferers) over negative results (acu-puncture doesn't help arthritis sufferers) when deciding which articles they will publish. While I will discuss this phenomenon and the reasons for its occurrence in much more detail in the next chapter (since it is an especially virulent source of bias in reviews of published research), it has to be briefly considered here because even single studies published in high-quality journals aren't immune from its effects.

For present purposes, suffice it to say that research journal editors, research sponsors, and researchers themselves prefer positive results over negative ones. This preference has been amusingly demonstrated by research methodologists who—with the blessings of the journals involved—sent out two versions of the same bogus article to journal reviewers.[7] The two study versions sent were identical except that one reported positive results and the other reported negative results.

So what happened? The positive study was considerably more likely to be accepted for publication.[8] Over time, this phenomenon means that positive studies tend to accumulate in the research record, a fact that naturally builds in a strong negative incentive for investigators to even try to publish a negative study.

Other methodologists of a more serious ilk have demonstrated that medical studies with statistically significant results are more likely to be published in the first place, to be published in prestigious journals, and even to be published more quickly.[9] Not to be left off this particular bandwagon, pharmaceutical sponsors of trials have been known to contribute their fair share to the problem by not allowing publication of negative findings and by threatening lawsuits against researchers who try to publish research showing that their drugs have higher incidences of side effects than their competitors' drugs.[10]

Again, we'll return to the issue of publication bias in Chapter 12, when we discuss systematic reviews of CAM research.

Statistical Bias, or Sir Ronald Fisher's Curse

As I've mentioned, people in my profession largely make their living by blessing the results of experiments as statistically significant or cursing them with the judgment that they are not statistically significant. While this judgment is exceedingly objective (and is now performed exclusively by computers), we owe a great deal of the popularity of the statistical significance concept to a statistician named Ronald A. Fisher.

The concept has a unique implication for us here since the decision whether a therapy is more effective than a placebo (i.e., positive) or not (i.e., negative) is based upon whether the computer deems the difference between the two to be statistically significant. The need for this convention emanates from two statistical facts of life: people differ from one another and nothing can be measured without some degree of error.

What this means in the context of a randomized, controlled trial is that if a deranged investigator were to randomly assign patients to two groups, both of which received an identical intervention under identical conditions for an identical period of time, the results obtained for these two groups would *not* be identical at the end of the study. One group would have improved slightly more (or would have degenerated slightly less) than the other—probably not by much, but the chances that the two groups would be absolutely identical for a reasonably sized trial would be about the same as those of your esteemed author being struck by a meteor next week.

Obviously, then, if there are always going to be differences between two groups following an experiment (and since every trial is different and every investigator has his or her own set of biases), some objective, agreed-upon standard is needed regarding which differences could be considered important and which could not. So about seventy years ago a very influential statistician named Sir Ronald Fisher suggested that a reasonable criterion for making this decision was to accept as significant any differences between groups that would occur by chance alone less than 5 percent of the time.

As one illustration of what this means, let's suppose that in a moment of weakness you bought a magic coin from a street vendor who promised you that, when flipped, it would land on heads more often than tails. Later, after suffering untold ridicule from friends and family, let's say that you decided to see if your coin would perform as promised.

Using our definition of statistical significance, this would mean that if you flipped your coin five times and it came up heads five times in a row, then your purchase should be regarded as an indicator of your financial acumen as opposed to the slightly more derogatory descriptors used by your boorish friends and uninformed family. Why? Because the probability of flipping a heads on the first trial would be ½ or 0.50, the probability of flipping two heads on the first two attempts would be ½ × ½ = 0.25, that of flipping three heads out of three tries would be 0.125, the chance of obtaining four heads in four attempts would be 0.0625, and the probability of getting five heads on the first five attempts would be ½ × ½ × ½ × ½ × ½ = 0.03125! Because this number is under 0.05, it meets our criterion of statistical significance. (It also means that if you were to repeat your five-flip experiment one hundred times, you would obtain five heads about three times.)

So while biostatisticians such as myself would assure you that your coin was indeed magical (some of the more conservative ones might propose an alternative explanation or two if they weren't too busy), perhaps this little example does illustrate the underlying meaning behind statistical significance. Perhaps it also illustrates why independent replication of research results is so important—and even why we can be told that hormone replacement therapy is beneficial one week and deadly the next.

While people have been bickering about Sir Ronald's advice for well over half a century now, it has become the de facto definition of real differences in experimental research. Differences that the computer (via the statistical analytic process) deems to have a probability level of less than or equal to 0.05 are designated as statistically significant. Those that the computer curses with a probability level of 0.06 (or higher) are designated as not significant. End of story.

Regardless of whether this is a sensible way to operate, it is in fact how things do operate in the world of science. And what it means is that for every twenty randomized, controlled trials conducted, one will be blessed as statistically significant when the differences between the experimental group (CAM therapy, in the present context) and the control group (or placebo here) in fact occurred by chance alone and were not real. What *this* means, in turn, given our current task of coming up with a definitive answer to the question of whether or not CAM therapies work better than a placebo, is that 5 percent of those trials judged to be positive really weren't. Of course, 5 percent isn't such a huge number, but it takes on added import when operating in conjunction with publication bias, which results in an additional bias toward accepting studies that have been erroneously assigned to this 5 percent category. And it becomes even more relevant when certain journals accept less than 10 percent of the studies submitted to them. It gets yet another unneeded boost when certain investigators allow bias (conscious or unconscious) to enter into their research.

TO THE RESCUE: QUALITY AND SIZE

Does the existence of all these sources of bias mean that we can't believe the results of published research reports? No, it doesn't, but it certainly means that we have to interpret the totality of the research in any given area with extreme caution. It also means that we must always keep these biases (due to the publication system, experimenters, scientific acculturation differences, and the 5 percent error rate associated with statistical significance) in mind. And it is even more important to realize that all of these factors, not to mention the legions of inferential artifacts already discussed, conspire to produce false positive results.

So, what's the bottom line? Is your esteemed author setting you up for a wimpy "maybe yes, maybe no" finale to our CAM-versus-placebo determination? No! Well, maybe. Regardless, I do feel an obligation to share the fact that the issues involved here are a bit more complicated than is realized by the people who discuss research findings on television, write about science in newspapers and magazines, try to sell you things based upon research evidence, and/or passionately advocate this or that CAM therapy. What almost inevitably occurs within the scientific literature for any therapy that attracts enough attention to warrant multiple clinical trials, CAM or otherwise, is a potpourri of initially conflicting results—most of them positive, some negative, and some merely equivocal.

What kind of CAM research should we consider acceptable to evaluate? Preferably:

High-quality, large (involving more than one research site if possible, which helps reduce experimenter bias), placebo-controlled RCTs verified by independent investigators (which is far and away our best protection against bias).

To put it another way, we could declare our criteria for acceptable evidence to be only those results from high-quality, large trials (say, with 100 patients or more per group) with independent replication. And by so doing, I could mercifully end this chapter and this book by authoritatively concluding that there is insufficient evidence that any CAM therapy is more effective than a credible placebo.

But as we've discussed, these are completely unrealistic criteria in an area such as CAM, where the difference between the most positive and most negative studies may reflect nothing more than a few centimeters on a self-reported visual analog scale. In addition, the investigators may not be that experienced; the vast majority of the studies are relatively old, small, or published in CAM journals that are more likely to have a bias toward publishing results that show that CAM works; and historically there hasn't been enough research funding to either conduct large studies or replicate past research efforts. In truth, especially in a field that is relatively new to serious scientific scrutiny, these criteria are unnecessarily stringent—especially for therapies that have few serious side effects associated with their use and for which only the deranged or the dangerously naive recommend their use as a first-line therapy in life-or-death situations.

So to be reasonable, I'll obviously have to relax the criteria a bit—although in so doing I will definitely increase the false positive rate of the evidence considered. Still, this is an acceptable trade-off here, since all I am really trying to do anyway is to provide a gestalt, painted in the very broadest of brushstrokes, of the evidence surrounding the equally broad question:

Is there acceptable evidence that any CAM therapy exerts any beneficial health effect over and above that attributable to the placebo effect and its epistemological cousins?

TOWARD A DEFINITION OF METHODOLOGICAL QUALITY

Here, then, are the criteria (alluded to in more general terms in Chapter 11) that I chose to decide whether or not a CAM trial could be considered as credible scientific evidence.

Criterion 1: The trial involves the random assignment of participants to both a CAM therapy and a credible placebo control group. In CAM (and especially given the specific issue under consideration), to produce credible results the trial must randomly assign participants to receive either the therapy being evaluated or a credible placebo that is indistinguishable from the real thing.

Criterion 2: The trial employs at least fifty participants per group. Small clinical trials simply cannot be counted on to produce reliable results. And while there are differences of opinion regarding the optimal size of a clinical trial, the minimum acceptable number of participants for trials that do not involve rare diseases (which CAM trials don't) or rarely occurring outcomes such as death (which they also don't) is no less than fifty participants per group.[11]

Criterion 3: The trial doesn't lose 25 percent or more of its participants over the course of the study. Regardless of how many people are enrolled in the trial, it is important that a large proportion of these patients do not drop out of the study before the intervention can be evaluated. Why? Because chances are the patients who drop out of a study are the ones who feel they aren't being helped, or who figure out that they have been assigned to the placebo group.

Criterion 4: The trial was published in a high-quality, prestigious, peer-reviewed journal. There are thousands of journals that publish medical research, which means that just about any positive trial that is written up can eventually, if its authors are persistent enough, get published somewhere regardless of its quality. The publishing journal takes on special importance in CAM research, however, since there are literally hundreds of CAM journals. And a homeopathy or acupuncture journal (whose subscription base is composed entirely of acupuncturists and homeopaths or devotees thereof) is far less likely to publish a trial that suggests acupuncture or homeopathy doesn't work than is a mainstream medical journal.

Fortunately, there is a relatively objective way to choose high-quality research journals, and that is to look at what is called "journal impact," which is based upon the number of times a given journal's research articles are cited by other researchers.[12] High-impact journals are also the most prestigious medical journals, which means that all medical researchers (CAM and conventional) aspire to have the results of their efforts published therein. Not coincidentally, they are also the types of journals that investigators' funding agencies prefer to see their clients publish in. The runaway leaders among general (non-disease-specific) American medical journals are the *New England Journal of Medicine* (*NEJM*) and the *Journal of the American Medical Association* (*JAMA*); hence, as described below, it is these two journals that I initially chose as optimal sources of high-quality CAM trials.

In support of these criteria, I now present three case studies, all of which were published in relatively high-quality, prestigious peer-reviewed journals but only one of which (the third) meets all four of our criteria (i.e., it was published in a high-quality journal, employed at least fifty patients per group, retained at least 75 percent of the participants throughout the course of the study, and employed a credible placebo control). While case studies such as these don't actually prove anything, I believe that they will provide a conceptual basis for understanding why all four criteria are important (especially employing a placebo control group) and convey a sense of the types of modern CAM studies that appear in high-quality journals (namely, studies employing very discrete interventions applied to very discrete medical conditions).

Example #1:

A Randomized (Non-Placebo-Controlled) Trial Contrasting a CAM Therapy with a Conventional Therapy Control

Title: "Effectiveness of Leech Therapy in Osteoarthritis of the Knee: A Randomized Controlled Trial"[13] (No, that's not a typo; it does say *leech*. Don't forget, this is CAM.)

Journal: *Annals of Internal Medicine* (While not quite in the class of *NEJM* and *JAMA*, the *Annals of Internal Medicine* is a very well-respected journal and has the third-highest impact score among American general medical journals.)

Background: Regretfully noting that "the application of medicinal leeches was widely practiced in ancient times, but their use has declined rapidly in Europe and America with the advent of modern surgery and pharmacology," these German researchers intrepidly set out to "evaluate the effectiveness of leech therapy for symptomatic relief of osteoarthritis of the knee." They correspondingly assigned twenty-four patients to receive four to six locally applied leeches and twenty-seven patients to receive a topically applied drug. (Note: this meets neither our group-size criterion nor our requirement of a randomized placebo control group—so what do you think? Will the results be positive or negative?)

Results: You're absolutely correct if you thought the results would be positive. After seven days, patients receiving leech therapy suffered less pain than those receiving the traditional therapy (topical diclofenac). Within four weeks this difference was no longer statistically significant, but the leech group still reported better function, less stiffness, and fewer overall symptoms.

Quiz: What important impediment to making causal inferences does this trial *not* control for? Is it (a) natural history, (b) aversion to absolutely disgusting life-forms, or (c) the placebo effect?

If you answered (a), you failed. Answering (b) is fairly understandable and simply means that you overlooked the fact that patients had to volunteer for this trial with the full knowledge that they were going to become quite intimate with this particular life form—the probability of which, prior to the advent of reality shows and my tenure at a CAM research center, I would have rated very low. If you answered (c), I consider myself a teacher of the Socratic class.

As I've mentioned before, people volunteer for trials that they believe might be able to help them. Few if any people volunteered for this trial because they had a burning desire to see if topical diclofenac would help them. If they wanted to ascertain this, it would take much less effort to go to their physician and request a prescription. Thus while the diclofenac might result in a very small placebo effect, the leeches would engender far and away the larger placebo response for this strange little sample of people.

If the investigators had consulted me. I would have suggested that they spend several years developing placebo leeches to adequately blind their patients. Or, if they were in a hurry, I might have suggested they try common garden-variety slugs attached with a drop of super-glue. (Which perhaps explains why I am not in more demand as a CAM consultant.)

Example #2:

A Randomized, Controlled Trial Contrasting a CAM Therapy with Another CAM Therapy

Title: "Randomized Trial Comparing Traditional Chinese Medical Acupuncture, Therapeutic Massage, and Self-Care Education for Chronic Low Back Pain"[14]

Journal: *Archives of Internal Medicine* (This is a step down the quality-journal food chain, but it still possesses the fourth-highest impact factor among general American medical journals.)

Background: The authors justify the study by citing two facts, neither of which I would disagree with. The first is that "back problems are among the most prevalent conditions afflicting Americans and one of the most common reasons for using complementary and alternative medical therapies." The second is that the research conducted to date assessing the efficacy of both acupuncture and massage for relieving back pain has been of abysmal quality. Unfortunately, in this particular study the investigators decided not to break with the tradition behind the second fact, since they randomly assigned 262 participants (a nice-sized trial) to one of three groups: acupuncture, massage, or self-care educational materials. An innovative feature of this trial was that all of the outcome data were collected over the telephone, a strategy that greatly reduced attrition but which prevented the collection of any physiological information.

Results: At the end of the treatment period, the massage group was superior to—you guessed it—the participants who received only some do-it-yourself instructions. A year later, the massage group was inexplicably superior to acupuncture but *not* to this self-help group.

What did the investigators conclude? "The results of this study suggest that massage is an effective short-term treatment for chronic low back pain, with benefits that persist for at least 1 year." More effective than what? At ten weeks, more effective than a group of people who received some handouts—which wouldn't be expected to carry much of a placebo wallop—and at one year (but not immediately) more effective than acupuncture. (Remember, one of the primary rationales used by the authors to justify this study in the first place was that there wasn't sufficient high-quality evidence to support acupuncture's effectiveness in reducing back pain.) Incredibly, they also concluded: "Because we did not include a 'no treatment' or 'standard care only' group, the results might underestimate the value of all 3 treatments." By now, I would hope that you would suspect that a less biased conclusion might have been: "Because we did not include a placebo group, the results might *overestimate* the value of all 3 treatments."

And since all journal editors require investigators to mention at least the primary limitations of the study, here is what our CAM researchers chose to identify: "The study's primary limitations are use of a single study site, the absence of a 'no treatment' or 'usual care' control group, restriction of the study to a single form of acupuncture (TCM), the possibility that acupuncturists and massage therapists were atypical, and use of protocols that excluded treatments often used by some TCM acupuncturists (e.g., herbs and oriental massage)." Still not a peep about the absence of a placebo group.

Quiz: Question 1: What's missing here? Is it (a) a homeopathy group, (b) leeches, or (c) a placebo control? Question 2: What did this study not control for? Is the answer (a) natural history, (b) aversion to absolutely disgusting life-forms, or (c) the placebo effect?

If you answered (c) to both questions, either my graduate students have been wrong all of these years about my teaching ability or I'm going to have to start rotating the location of the correct answers soon. Since there is no placebo group, there is no way to determine whether any statistically significant results favoring one or both of the CAM treatments are due to treatment or to the placebo effect. We've already established that some placebos are more effective than others (in fact, a few years later one of the authors here actually conducted the study cited in Chapter 8 that definitively demonstrated this fact), so why couldn't some therapies be more effective than others solely because they produced more potent placebo effects? Furthermore, by putting in a group that simply receives self-care materials, the investigators are contrasting two CAM treatments to a very, very weak control group that would not be expected to elicit much of a placebo effect at all. (And whose participants undoubtedly felt disappointed, if not downright cheated, when they were told that the computer had decided that they would receive a few handouts instead of free massage or acupuncture sessions.)

For any readers who may someday choose to evaluate research evidence on their own, my advice is to focus on the report's methods and procedure section (where such issues as blinding, random assignment, sample size, and attrition are discussed) and its results section (where the authors will note what was and was not statistically significant) but to pretty much ignore the investigators' discussion/conclusions section. It is in that last section that the authors, if it is their wont, will try to put a spin on their data. And while this may seem to be rather pejorative advice, it is actually the tack taken by researchers who conduct systematic reviews, which is one advantage that genre of research has over the interpretation of individual trials—and which in turn is why I have devoted the next chapter to considering systematic reviews of the effectiveness of CAM therapies.

Example #3:

A Randomized, Controlled Trial Contrasting a CAM Therapy with a Credible CAM Placebo Group

Title: "Effects of Magnetic vs. Sham-Magnetic Insoles on Plantar Heel Pain"[15]

Journal: *Journal of the American Medical Association*

Background: The article begins by talking about how rapidly the use of magnets for pain relief has increased in the past ten years (which is true of almost all CAM therapies) and about the fact that an estimated $500 million on magnets is being spent annually in the United States alone. Some studies have shown that magnets work to a small extent, but slightly more studies have found that they do not. (Which, incidentally, is why we are focusing on high-quality research in this book.) The present study was therefore designed to "assess the effectiveness of bipolar static magnets in insoles for the treatment of plantar [on the sole of the foot] heel pain." A total of 101 patients were randomly assigned to one of two groups. The experimental group received a commercially available magnetic insole, and the control group received an identical insole except that the implanted metallic substance was not magnetized. At baseline (prior to receiving their insoles) and at both four and eight weeks, all participants were administered pain assessments. (Note that all four of our quality criteria were met.)

Results: As always in trials such as this (which are substantially impacted by the placebo effect and its degenerate family—natural history, the Hawthorne effect, and so forth), both groups reported significantly less pain over time, although there was absolutely no difference at four and eight weeks between the experimental and placebo groups. The authors therefore concluded: "Although many claims have been made regarding the therapeutic use of magnets, our outcomes showed static magnets to be ineffective in the treatment of plantar heel pain."

This was a very well-designed, placebo-controlled trial, and while it might have been possible for participants to have identified which group they had been assigned to by passing a ferrous metal object over their insoles, such an action would have conspired to produce false positive effects rather than false negative ones.[16] Since the results were negative, this obviously wasn't a problem. It does, however, illustrate how difficult it is to construct reasonably credible placebos for CAM therapies.

Quiz: Why do you think these investigators didn't emphasize the fact that both of their interventions (real and sham magnets) resulted in decreased pain? Is it that (a) they didn't understand the effects that regression to the mean and the placebo effect can have on research involving pain, (b) they weren't properly trained CAM researchers, or (c) they really wanted to investigate the effect of a different intervention on heel pain but their participants kept stepping on the leeches? Quite frankly, I'm not sure about the answer to this one myself. But let's just go with (c), since that usually seems to be the correct answer.

An Important Concession

These three articles shared some interesting similarities and differences. All three were randomized, controlled trials, none witnessed a significant dropout rate, and all were published in well-recognized U.S. medical journals. Two were positive and one was negative. Not coincidentally, the one producing negative results employed both a credible placebo as its control group and at least fifty participants per group.

I have no doubt that if all the CAM trials published in all of the non-CAM research journals were compared using just these two simple criteria, this same pattern would occur at least 90 percent of the time. Since I haven't taken the time to make this comparison, and given my age I don't have the time to make it, I therefore happily concede that the preponderance of evidence for trials evaluating CAM therapies in relation to conventional therapies or to no treatment at all probably favors CAM therapies simply because RCTs are very good at documenting placebo effects and other inferential artifacts. On the other side of the coin, properly performed RCTs are abysmally poor at documenting the superiority of CAM effects in comparison to placebos—either because they don't exist or because they are exceedingly rare.

HIGH-QUALITY CAM TRIALS PUBLISHED IN HIGH-QUALITY MEDICAL JOURNALS, JANUARY 2000–FEBRUARY 2007

Now let's turn to a broader survey of results from other CAM trials. I chose the year 2000 as my beginning point for two reasons: intuitively it sounded good because it was the beginning of a new millennium, and methodologically it seemed reasonable because trials that began showing up at this point in time should have had access to the CON-SORT statement.[17] I also decided, at least originally, to go through only the CAM placebo-controlled trials published in *JAMA* and *NEJM* for the past seven years as of this writing, February 6, 2007. As mentioned, both journals are head and shoulders above most other medical journals with respect to quality and influence. Both are also subscribers to the CON-SORT statement, which basically means that they attempt to publish only research that adequately controls for the sources of bias that have been discussed up to this point, by authors who are transparent about how they went about controlling for these sources of bias. Said another way, these are the two journals in which almost all clinically oriented medical researchers aspire to publish their work. I might also mention an irony: it was these two journals that brought CAM research into the scientific spotlight by publishing the Harvard CAM surveys (noted in Chapter 1) that purported to prove that visits to CAM providers exceeded visits to primary care physicians. So because just about every CAM research article cites these two surveys, and just about every public statement emanating from the National Center for Complementary and Alternative Medicine cites at least one of them, it is probably fair to say that these two journals helped launch the modern CAM research era.

In any case, beyond publication in a high-quality journal such as *JAMA* or *NEJM*, the only restrictions that I used to select the studies in this survey were the three other criteria identified earlier: that is, the presence of a randomly assigned placebo group, at least fifty participants per group, and a dropout rate of less than 25 percent. My method of finding these articles was also quite straightforward: I simply examined all of the articles published in the two journals over the time period in question.

Journal of the American Medical Association (*JAMA*)

Ten trials meeting the above-mentioned criteria were published by *JAMA* during this period. For each trial I have included an icon that indicates a positive (+) or negative (−) conclusion regarding the effectiveness of the therapy in question, based upon the authors' own assessments, which are provided in the form of direct quotes.

1 −

Herbal (Guggulipid) for High Cholesterol

"Guggulipid did not appear to improve levels of serum cholesterol over the short term in this population of adults with hypercholesterolemia."[18]

2 –

Acupuncture for Cocaine Addiction

"Within the clinical context of this study, acupuncture was not more effective than a [non-acupuncture-related] needle insertion or relaxation control in reducing cocaine use."[19]

3 –

Clover Extract for the Treatment of Menopause Symptoms

"Neither supplement [Promensil and Rimostil were contrasted to a placebo] had a clinically important effect on hot flashes or other symptoms of menopause."[20]

4 –

Chelation Therapy for Heart Disease

"There is no evidence to support a beneficial effect of chelation therapy in patients with ischemic heart disease, stable angina, and a positive treadmill test for ischemia."[21]

5 –

St. John's Wort for Depression

"In this study, St. John's wort was not effective for treatment of major depression."[22]

6 –

St. John's Wort for Depression: The Sequel

"The study fails to support the efficacy of *H. perforatum* [St. John's wort] in moderately severe depression."[23]

7 –

Ginkgo for Memory

"These data suggest that when taken following the manufacturer's instructions, ginkgo provides no measurable benefit in memory or related cognitive function in adults with healthy cognitive function."[24]

8 –

Magnets for Heel Pain

"Static bipolar magnets embedded in cushioned shoe insoles do not provide additional benefit for subjective plantar heel pain when compared with nonmagnetic insoles."[25]

This was the study used as a more detailed example earlier in the chapter.

9 –

Echinacea for Upper Respiratory Tract Infections in Children

"*Echinacea purpurea*, as dosed in this study, was not effective in treating upper respiratory infection symptoms in patients 2 to 11 years old, and its use was associated with an increased risk of rash."[26]

10 –

Acupuncture for Patients with Migraine

> "Acupuncture was no more effective than sham acupuncture in reducing migraine headaches although both interventions were more effective than a waiting list control."[27]

Of course both were more effective than a waiting list (which means no treatment) control—they were both placebos. The *JAMA* editors allowed the primary authors, who were affiliated with German CAM centers, to call the placebo control group an intervention and to equivocate mightily: "The lack of differences between acupuncture and sham acupuncture in our study indicates that point location and other aspects considered relevant for acupuncture did not make a difference." The bottom line is clear, however: acupuncture is no more effective than a placebo.

Is it just me, or do you detect a trend here? Ten trials (even ten high-quality ones) certainly aren't enough to answer our original question, but it is interesting that all ten failed to find any evidence supporting the superiority of a CAM therapy over a placebo.

The New England Journal of Medicine

Alas, despite getting the entire CAM field off to a running start in 1993 (or perhaps in penitence for it), *NEJM* published only four CAM trials meeting our criteria during the seven-year interval.

11 –

Chelation Therapy for Children Exposed to Lead

> "Treatment with succimer lowered blood lead levels but did not improve scores on test of cognition, behavior, or neuropsychological function in children with blood lead levels below 45 μg

per deciliter...chelation therapy is not indicated for children with these blood levels."[28]

Succimer is an oral lead-chelating drug that, in this trial, briefly lowered the children's lead levels but to such a small degree that little measurable cognitive benefit could be expected.

12 –

Echinacea Treatment for Experimentally Induced Rhinovirus Infection

"The results of this study indicate that extracts of *E. angustifolia* root, either alone or in combination, do not have clinically significant effects on infection with a rhinovirus or on the clinical illness that results from it."[29]

13 –

Saw Palmetto for Benign Prostatic Hyperplasia

"In this study, saw palmetto did not improve symptoms or objective measures of benign prostatic hyperplasia."[30]

14 –

Glucosamine, Chondroitin Sulfate, and the Two in Combination for Painful Knee Osteoarthritis

"Glucosamine and chondroitin sulfate alone or in combination did not reduce pain effectively in the overall group of patients with osteoarthritis of the knee."[31]

The Bottom Line, and a Caveat

The score is 14–0 so far for placebo versus CAM. However, as should be apparent from the discussion in Chapter 1, definitions of what is and is not considered CAM vary. As a result, I excluded from my search some therapies or procedures that some people would consider CAM but which I do not. For example, I didn't include hyperbaric oxygen as a CAM therapy in this book, although I'm sure that some people would. (There was one such study in *NEJM* during this period involving the use of hyperbaric oxygen in cases of carbon monoxide poisoning, but since it too was negative, its inclusion wouldn't have changed the results.) And as I mentioned in Chapter 1, I also made a decision early on not to include vitamin or mineral supplementation as CAM therapies, although according to some definitions they do qualify when they are prescribed to treat or prevent specific diseases. I did notice several such studies in my searches, as illustrated by the following, which tends to be typical of such studies published in these two journals.

Vitamin E and Multivitamin-Mineral Supplements for Acute Respiratory Tract Infections

"Neither daily multivitamin supplementation at physiological dose nor 200 mg of vitamin E showed a favorable effect on incidence and severity of acute respiratory tract infections in well-nourished noninstitutionalized elderly individuals. Instead we observed adverse effects of vitamin E on illness severity."[32]

BACK TO THE DRAWING BOARD: *ANNALS OF INTERNAL MEDICINE*

At the risk of suffering a host of slings and arrows from my peers, I decided to abandon my original plan and expand my search to some more journals. (Normally in research we are taught to specify our research plan in advance and stick to it.) I therefore chose the two most prestigious general scientific journals in existence (which are *Science* and *Nature*) and the third most prestigious medical journal, the *Annals of Internal Medicine,* which is a high-impact, high-quality medical journal that ascribes to the CONSORT statement.

I felt sort of good about these new journal choices since they had the potential to add a different perspective to my search. *Science* and *Nature* do not normally publish clinical trials, although the former published some of the placebo trials involving brain scans I discussed earlier and the latter published one of the most famous CAM-type studies of all time a couple of decades ago, purporting to show that exposing our children to Mozart would make them smarter. (Alas, it couldn't be replicated.) And while I never saw this intervention referred to as a CAM therapy, it is definitely of the "man bites dog and several other animals" genre, with which both of these journals occasionally spice their more mundane offerings.

As for the *Annals of Internal Medicine,* it occurred to me that some of my CAM critics might argue that my choosing only *JAMA* and *NEJM* may have stacked the deck against finding high-quality CAM trials. Personally, I doubt that these journals are biased against CAM, since large capitalistic research enterprises *like* to publish research articles that will interest their readers and generate press coverage in the popular media. And "man bites dog" or "homeopathy better than insulin for diabetics" will get them a lot more of this coverage (and result in more new subscribers) than the converse.

There is no question, however, that the *Annals* has a very positive editorial attitude favoring CAM, since this journal chose to publish an entire *series* of CAM articles—a decision the editors argued "reflects the *Annals'* continuing interest in the practice of medicine in the broadest sense."[33] Unfortunately, none of the articles that the specially appointed editor, a director of one of the original NIH-funded CAM research centers, chose to publish were placebo-controlled trials that met our quality criteria. (I should mention that it was the *Annals* that chose to publish the above-presented leech study.)

In any event, during the seven-year interval I found no reasonably sized, placebo-controlled trials in *Nature* or *Science* and only four in the

Annals. The first trial, which evaluated the effectiveness of echinacea in treating the common cold, also turned out to be negative despite the fact, mentioned in the report, that numerous studies—mostly German, incidentally—had addressed echinacea's botanical, chemical, and pharmacologic characteristics and clinical effects.

15 –

Treatment of the Common Cold with Unrefined Echinacea: A Randomized Double-Blind, Placebo-Controlled Trial

> "Compared to placebo, unrefined echinacea provided no detectable benefit or harm in these college students who had the common cold."[34]

I was able to locate three other CAM trials that met my criteria.

16 –

Acupuncture for Chronic Mechanical Neck Pain

> "Acupuncture reduced neck pain and produced a statistically, but not clinically, significant effect compared with placebo. The beneficial effects of acupuncture for pain may be due to both nonspecific and specific effects."[35]

The authors reported having specified prior to conducting the study what they would consider to be positive results, and the difference they obtained was considerably less than this (only 6 on a 1–100 scale). Because of the authors' obvious integrity in setting a high target for what they would consider positive and then in reporting that original target, a transparency I greatly admire and which, at least based upon my five-year experience in the field, is quite rare, I almost hate to count this as a negative study. This is, however, a typical price that scientists pay for conducting high-quality trials and reporting their results honestly.

17 –

Acupuncture and Knee Osteoarthritis: A Three-Armed Randomized Trial

"No statistically significant difference was observed between TCA [traditional Chinese acupuncture] and sham acupuncture suggesting that the observed difference could be due to placebo effects, differences in intensity of provider contact, or a physiological effect of needling regardless of whether it is done according to TCA principles."[36]

The third arm was physician care alone. As is usual for CAM authors from Germany, the authors could not quite accept the fact that their data definitely demonstrated the presence of a placebo effect for acupuncture.

18 –

Black Cohosh and Multibotanicals for Vasomotor Menopausal Symptoms

"Black cohosh used in isolation, or as part of a mulitbotanical regimen, shows little potential as an important therapy for relief of vasomotor symptoms."[37]

I should mention that the *Annals* did publish several trials comparing CAM therapies to conventional ones (such as manual therapy versus physical therapy and usual care, and one comparing acupuncture and massage with treatment as usual), but they lacked placebo controls and so their positive results in favor of CAM are neither surprising nor credible.

In Desperation: *Archives of Internal Medicine*

Partially because I never suspected a complete shutout and partially because I had a lingering fear that no one would believe the results I found in the journals just mentioned, I decided to keep searching until I could find one positive high-quality trial published in a reputable American journal. (If nothing else, you will remember that statistical theory, à la Sir Ronald Fisher, predicts that we should find one positive result out of twenty if only random chance were operating.) Toward this end, I selected the *Archives of Internal Medicine* in the desperate hope that I would find something and not be suspected of bias myself. This is the journal that, as described in the second case study above, allowed its CAM investigators so much leeway in their statement of limitations that they weren't required to mention that their CAM-versus-CAM-versus-nothing study didn't include a placebo control. The other four studies I found did at least include that.

19 –

Echinacea purpurea *Therapy for the Treatment of the Common Cold: A Randomized, Double-Blind, Placebo-Controlled Trial*

"Some studies have concluded that Echinacea effectively reduces the symptoms and duration of the common cold. We were unable to replicate such findings."[38]

20 –

Acupuncture in Patients with Chronic Low Back Pain: A Randomized, Controlled Trial

"Acupuncture was more effective in improving pain than no acupuncture treatment in patients with chronic low back pain, whereas there were no significant differences between acupuncture and minimal acupuncture."[39]

Obviously, we know that there is such a thing as a placebo effect.

21 · −

Acupuncture for Subacute Stroke Rehabilitation: A Sham-Controlled, Subject- and Accessor-Blind Randomized Trial

"Acupuncture is not superior to sham treatment for recovery in activities of daily living and health-related quality of life after stroke, although there may be a limited effect on leg function in more severely affected patients."[40]

In RCT terminology, the latter finding is called a subgroup analysis and isn't given a lot of credence because it is often possible to find that the treatment works for some group of patients on some outcome by chance alone if the investigations conduct enough analyses. In methodological terminology, it is called a "fishing expedition."

22 +

Cholesterol-Lowering Effect of a Theaflavin-Enriched Green Tea Abstract: A Randomized, Controlled Trial

"The theaflavin-enriched green tea extract we studied is an effective adjunct to a low-saturated-fat diet to reduce LDL-C in hypercholesterolemic adults and is well tolerated."[41]

At last, a positive CAM trial. So what if over half of the sample drank at least one cup of tea a day anyway, and 27 percent of these drank more than five cups per day? And so what if, as indicated in the article's footnote, the principal investigator was a consultant for Nashai Biotech, LLC, whose principal product (at least the one that popped up immediately when I accessed the company's Web site) happens to be this very product? So what if another author of this *Archives* paper was a vice president of Nashai Biotech, and yet another was its chief science officer? We finally have a positive placebo-controlled trial that involved more than fifty participants and that had an attrition rate below 25 percent! Perhaps finding one positive trial has helped me maintain my credibility; it has at least provided Sir Ronald Fisher's 5 percent rule with an unneeded validation.

NEEDED: ANOTHER APPROACH

Even with our expanded search, twenty-two large, high-quality trials are hardly a sufficient basis upon which to conclude that CAM therapies are nothing more than placebos, even if the score is 21–1.[42] Of course, we could keep expanding our search from journal to journal until we reached something like, oh, the *French Journal of Homeopathic Research* or even the *Proceedings of the Beijing People's Acupuncture Society*, but the results of this extended exercise would be predictable. As it is, limiting our search to moderately sized studies that retain at least 75 percent of their participants and insisting upon the presence of a randomized placebo control group means that we must bypass most such journals and therefore miss at least 95 percent of CAM trials. But if we were to relax our criteria and move down the journal food chain (which in effect waters down the peer review process and its incumbent insistence upon quality), we will gradually find more and more positive trials until we arrive at the real bottom-feeders, where everything will be positive.

Our results so far indicate that when high-quality, placebo-controlled trials in high-quality, selective journals are considered, the preponderance of the evidence suggests that CAM therapies do not produce beneficial effects over and above those that can be explained by the placebo effect. But the bottom line is that there just isn't enough of this sort of evidence to arrive at a truly convincing conclusion about this question.

Fortunately, there is another very impressive source of evidence that we haven't yet considered for making sense of the voluminous CAM trials, one that doesn't completely ignore quality or embrace bias. While this particular method treats all research journals as though they were created equally (which, trust me, they aren't) and it doesn't completely ignore trials that employ non-placebo controls (which I personally believe is a mistake), it does factor quality (including the presence or absence of non-placebo controls) and trial size into its bottom-line conclusions. This method, the end results of which are called systematic reviews or meta-analyses, suffers from one other, huge disadvantage: it elevates publication bias to an art form—to a point, in fact, that some credible research methodologists and many trialists discount this type of evidence completely. Still, while I have moved toward their point of view over the years as well, it is not a universally accepted position and, given the dearth of high-quality individual CAM trials available, I would certainly be remiss if I did not explore systematic reviews as a rich source of evidence. That is the focus of the next chapter.

CHAPTER TWELVE

What High-Quality Systematic Reviews Reveal About CAM[1]

I've already mentioned the fact that there are thousands of research journals and archives containing the results of hundreds of thousands of research trials. In the past few decades an exceedingly creative tool has evolved to help us make sense of this embarrassment of riches. In 1976, a research methodologist named Gene V. Glass published a paper unremarkably titled "Primary, Secondary, and Meta-analysis of Research," in which he proposed a new approach for dealing with the results of multiple trials designed to evaluate the same interventions.[1]

Proposing something is a lot easier than doing it, so Glass and his wife, Mary Lee Smith, proceeded to illustrate this approach by assessing several hundred trials surrounding two of the most frequently researched areas in psychiatry and education—all of which were designed to answer two apparently simple questions: (1) Does psychotherapy work? (2) Do students taught in small classes learn more than students taught in large classes?

At first glance these may seem like relatively obvious questions. Of course psychotherapy helps people, and anyone who knows anything about education knows that children learn more in small classes than in large ones. The trouble was that despite the plethora of studies evaluating both issues, their results weren't that easy to interpret. There were many reasons for this, but the two most important were that the vast majority of these studies were of abysmally poor quality and that there was no objective way of boiling down the evidence from so many studies with so many conflicting results into a simple yes/no, "it works/it doesn't work" answer. A reviewer could always count up the number of positive results and compare this figure to the number of negative results, but if this were done in the 1970s, the answer to at least the class size question would have been a definitive no. Yet everyone and everyone's grandmother knew that small classes were better than large ones, so something was obviously wrong.

I won't bore you with the technicalities of how the researchers solved this problem, but their approach had two crucially innovative tenets:

1. The researchers insisted on very systematic search procedures (hence the term "systematic review") to find *all* of the trials that had been completed. This commonsense strategy basically transformed the research review into a scientific strategy that could be replicated by other researchers.

2. The results of these individual studies were then used in much the same way that statisticians use results from individual trial participants. In other words, instead of pooling and analyzing the outcome results obtained from psychotherapy patients in a single study (or from students taking tests in large classrooms compared to small ones), as is done in clinical trials, the researchers pooled the results of entire trials and analyzed these pooled results to ascertain statistical significance or lack of significance. What did they find? Both systematic reviews (also called meta-analyses) produced definitive yes answers to their respective research questions.[2]

Over the years that followed, this approach has evolved somewhat in medicine. Today, instead of giving equal weight to high- and low-quality trials, we generally only consider randomized, controlled trials, and we attempt to arrive at a bottom-line conclusion based upon these trials by factoring in such characteristics as study size and methodological quality, among other things.[3] To facilitate this process, an incredible organization has come into existence devoted to the task of synthesizing the results of multiple trials into definitive answers regarding which therapies do and do not work.

THE COCHRANE COLLABORATION

Spearheaded by Iain Chalmers, a British physician and research methodologist, the Cochrane Collaboration (named after a famous statistician, Dr. Archibald Cochrane) is surely the most remarkable research institution in existence. (If I were in charge of writing the history of science, in fact, Iain Chalmers and Gene Glass would have prominent places reserved for them by the time I finished with the second half of the twentieth century.) A loosely but thoughtfully organized band of dedicated professionals from all over the world set out in 1993 to collect, synthesize, and evaluate all existing knowledge relevant to medical care. More than six thousand individuals from over sixty countries around the world now contribute to the achievement of this extremely ambitious objective. It is supported by more than 650 international organizations, including health service providers, research funding agencies, departments of health, international organizations, industry, and universities.[4]

The organization's main product and most impressive accomplishment is the Cochrane Database of Systematic Reviews (the Cochrane Collaboration prefers the term "systematic review" to "meta-analysis"), and it is available electronically via the Cochrane Library. Several hundred reviews are added each year to the database, which as of this writing (May 2007) now contains approximately 3,100 completed reviews. Their purpose is quite simple: to provide reliable reviews of evidence that are up-to-date and easily accessible to people making decisions regarding medical treatment (physicians and consumers).

I chose this database to expand our evidence for two very explicit reasons besides its sheer size. First, the Cochrane Collaboration is practically obsessed with producing high-quality, unbiased reviews, given that quality and the avoidance of bias are as important in conducting reviews of trials as they are in conducting the trials themselves. In fact, the organization will not add a review to its database that does not comply with its voluminous set of regulations and safeguards, the most important of which from our perspective is that the quality of the trials must be factored into a succinct, bottom-line conclusion. Second, while organized medicine might be susceptible to accusations of bias toward CAM, the Cochrane Collaboration is not. The entire reason for this organization's existence is to provide the public and the medical profession with unbiased assessments of what works and what does not work, and it takes this mission very seriously.

What I did, therefore, was go through the entire database in search of systematic reviews involving CAM therapies. I was a little more successful in my literature search this time around, finding ninety-eight reviews of therapies that involved at least two trials. The therapies themselves ranged from acupuncture and artichoke leaf extract to ultrasound and yoga, although upon examination the yoga review had to be dropped since it involved only one trial.

Adopting the two-trial minimum as my only criterion in selecting these reviews meant that I would have to abandon the more stringent quality standards employed in Chapter 1 ˉ and instead open myself up to the full array of studies that the Cochrane Collaboration aspires to include—that is, all studies conducted to evaluate the effectiveness of a treatment, be they large or small, published in high-impact journals or obscure ones, placebo-controlled or not, competently or incompetently run, conducted a few decades before or within a few years after the CONSORT statement appeared. This isn't to say that Cochrane reviewers do not take the size or the quality of a trial into consideration in reaching their bottom-line conclusion. They do. Their prime directive, however, is to locate and evaluate all of the evidence surrounding the efficacy of any given treatment, be it the farthest-out CAM therapy conceivable or the latest and greatest surgical procedure. Thus, given our objectives here,

I will occasionally interject a brief commentary on some of these reviews, especially with respect to the absence of decent-sized, placebo-controlled trials.

A HUGE, UGLY FLY IN THE OINTMENT

If this reads like an unabashed testimonial for the Cochrane Collaboration, it is. I have always greatly admired the seminal meta-analytic work of Iain Chalmers (along with his colleagues Murray Enkin and Marc Keirse) in pregnancy and childbirth; containing hundreds of individual meta-analyses, their review is, I believe, one of the most impressive scholarly achievements in history.[5] I have also published a special issue on the Cochrane Collaboration in the journal for which I serve as editor, *Evaluation and the Health Professions;* the special issue was edited by Mike Clarke, director of the U.K. Cochrane Centre, and I was most pleased when Chalmers agreed to contribute the issue's lead article.

Still, all meta-analyses, while far and away the best strategy that we have for synthesizing research evidence, are especially susceptible to one of the problems that I discussed in the previous chapter. It is a problem that, in my opinion, is so virulent for systematic reviews of published research that it may well constitute an insurmountable obstacle.

The problem, of course, is publication bias, which, the reader will remember, is a documented tendency for journal editors and their reviewers to prefer to publish positive results over negative ones and for investigators themselves to be less likely even to write up negative (or equivocal) results. While some reviewers attempt to minimize this bias by systematically locating all of the trials surrounding a given therapy, published and unpublished, the reality of the situation is that it is almost impossible to locate any substantial number of unpublished randomized, controlled trials for any given combination of medical condition and therapy. What this means, in turn, is that positive trials tend to populate systematic reviews, while negative trials tend to populate their investigators' file drawers.

To achieve a better conceptual understanding of how this phenomenon occurs, how it contributes to false positive results, and what its implications are, it may be helpful to consider a few concrete examples.

Scenario 1. Let's say that two scientists conduct the same experiment. Dr. A gets positive results, while Dr. B gets negative results. While we don't know which investigator was correct, we do know that Dr. A's study is more likely to be published, which means that probably no one will ever hear about Dr. B's. Such an occurrence is understandable from several perspectives, the most important of which is emotional in nature. Journal editors are more interested in publishing a new finding that describes something that can help people than in publishing one describing something that does them no good. By default this preference consigns unpublished studies almost to the same fate as research that was never conducted. While this is a shame for Dr. B, it has more serious implications for the scientific databases that constitute the raw materials for systematic reviews. Simply put, the databases are uneven in their holdings and are weighted toward positive findings because more studies like Dr. A's were published than were studies like Dr. B's. Thus even if the positive studies were as likely to be correct as the negative ones, there would be a greater proportion of false positive than false negative results winding up in systematic reviews due to publication bias. No one knows the extent of this problem, but we do know that when a team of reviewers collects all the published studies addressing a given issue, at the very least they (through no fault of their own) will wind up with an unrepresentatively large number of false positive trials. This in turn will inevitably result in a larger proportion of false positive systematic reviews than is scientifically warranted.

Scenario 2. Now consider two different scientists. Investigator C is a principled, careful professional, whereas investigator D will do anything to put a positive spin on his or her data, from selective reporting of only the positive aspects of the study to outright fabrication of data. While I'm not a student of motivations or incentives, I believe that some behavior like that of investigator D is due to the investigator being so convinced that the data *should* be positive that he or she actually believes that "correcting" it is preferable to publishing an erroneous result. Regardless of the "why" of their differences, investigator D will not produce many negative studies, so his or her research is much more likely to be published than the principled, carefully done research of investigator C.

Ultimately in science there are severe penalties for not getting one's research published. While most academics would recoil at this statement, the truth of the matter is that research (especially medical research) is a business. And while scientists are not paid for each research article they write, they are very definitely rewarded on the basis of their published research in terms of tenure, promotion, and pay raises. In addition, almost all investigators (especially in the health fields) depend upon grant money to be able to conduct research in the first place, not to mention the fact that these grants constitute a substantial proportion of their actual salaries. To make matters even stickier, the organizations that fund research (be they pharmaceutical companies or, to some extent, even governmental agencies such as the NIH) prefer positive results, which in turn produce yet another tangible incentive to generate positive results.

Why? Because behind these funding sources, as in journal publishing, are human beings with the fallibly human tendency to prefer good news over bad. Political and economic factors come into play as well. Legislators are not especially interested in telling their constituents that they support agencies that have discovered a plethora of interventions (be they drugs or CAM therapies) that do not help people—any more than pharmaceutical CEOs enjoy proudly announcing to their stockholders that the new drug the company has spent the last five years and $50 million developing has been definitively demonstrated to be worthless.

Scenario 3. The final scenario is not as well known as the other two, even among professionals who make their living conducting clinical trials. It involves a situation in which an investigator is personally identified with a specific therapy or clinical strategy. Once such individuals become well established, they often begin to derive a significant portion of their salaries (and, perhaps equally important, a portion of their self-esteem) from giving invited lectures to organizations of like-minded individuals. What this means is that such clinicians (or those who aspire to be in this situation) will be more reluctant to publish research that might be met with disfavor (or disbelief) among their colleagues. If such an individual is unfortunate enough to conduct a study so negative that its results can't be spun into something positive (and if the investigator is too ethical to alter the data), then he or she would have a very real public relations problem and a definite incentive not to publish the results at all.

While not publishing may sound (and ultimately is) unethical, it is also understandable and may be completely unconscious. Writing and publishing a research article is an onerous task and requires a degree of motivation to complete. When that motivation disappears or becomes negative in nature, the task often simply does not get accomplished.

Thus if a substantial number of investigators are motivated for personal or professional reasons not to take the time to write up the results of negative trials (or if they are simply *less* motivated to spend the time and energy necessary to do so), then the most careful and stringently conducted systematic Cochrane review imaginable will produce biased results, since it is based on reports whose positive findings encountered fewer, if any, barriers to publication. And a collection of ninety-eight systematic reviews such as I have identified will produce a certain percentage that are positive due to publication bias alone. What this percentage is, unfortunately, no one knows.

ANOTHER PRETTY LARGE FLY

A problem encountered in all placebo-controlled trials involves the credibility of the placebo itself. Even in drug trials that have the luxury of formulating a pill or capsule that is practically indistinguishable in taste, smell, and appearance from the active drug, research participants often guess which treatment they are in by the end of a trial.[6] But as we have discussed, this is even more likely to happen in trials of certain CAM therapies, for which developing a believable placebo procedure is difficult at best. Thus even the best sham acupuncture needles don't penetrate the skin, and—let's face it—it's not hard to know what does and does not penetrate our skin. Acupuncture-like electrical stimulation (such as transcutaneous electrical nerve stimulation, or TENS), another commonly used CAM treatment for pain, is a second case in point. On the surface TENS investigators appear to have come up with a very creative placebo, consisting of a electical stimulation machine that blinks and occasionally buzzes but does not deliver electrical stimulation. However, most of us are also sensitive enough to know when electricity is coursing through our bodies, especially when the current is sometimes strong enough to cause minor muscle contractions. Even some CAM therapies that seem tailor-made for placebo trials can be problematic, such as certain herbal formulations; in the words of one group of Cochrane reviewers, "ensuring participants are blind to their treatment is especially difficult when herbal medicines are given in a liquid form … which can be readily seen, smelt, and tasted … this obviously raises questions of the placebo effect on these results." (See review 37 below.) What does this mean? By now you should probably know the answer: inadequate blinding of participants translates into a source of positive bias in individual studies because the treatment group receives more of a placebo boost than the placebo group. And if this occurs in individual studies, it will surface in systematic reviews of them.

RELATED FLIES

Therapist-Initiated Placebo Effects

As we've already discussed, practitioners themselves are capable of unconsciously communicating their expectations and beliefs to their patients.[7] And since the practitioners of a number of CAM therapies (e.g., acupuncture, chiropractic, and massage) can't be blinded, it is almost a certainty that these therapists increase the placebo effect in the intervention group and decrease it in the control group. Out of sheer compassion I won't reiterate the effect that this has on RCTs and systematic reviews investigating the effectiveness of these therapies, except to say that they all begin with a positive placebo boost.

Trial Size

Although Cochrane reviews take the size of a trial into consideration when they weigh the available evidence, small trials create a unique challenge for systematic reviews. They are confounded with several problems in a rather complex manner, leading to what are called "small-study effects."[8] These are illustrated by the following two scenarios.

Scenario 1: a small, high-quality trial producing negative results. In this case, let's assume that a carefully conducted small trial has produced negative results. (All things being equal, in fact, it is a well-documented statistical fact that small trials should be more likely to produce negative results than positive ones.)[9] We already know that it will have some difficulty getting published—either because journal editors favor positive trials or because the trial's investigators don't try as hard as they might to get their study results published: perhaps they fear publication bias, or they have a distaste for negative trials themselves, or they're subject to professional/business pressures against publishing these negative results. Added to these various possibilities is the fact that small trials involve less effort and expense to conduct and hence may not have a funding agency advocating for the publication of their results. Whatever the case, we have another example of negative results being underrepresented in systematic reviews.

Scenario 2: a small, poor-quality trial producing positive results. In this scenario, we have a sloppily run (and therefore potentially biased) small trial that, as we've discussed, is more likely to produce positive results because of these factors. It, however, has publication bias working for it, so it is more likely to be accepted for publication by journal reviewers. Its authors also have more incentive to publish it, since a positive small trial provides an excellent case for convincing a funding agency to fund a larger trial.

In fact, almost all large funding agencies, especially the NIH, require investigators to provide evidence of successful preliminary studies before committing the million-plus dollars necessary to fund a large RCT. This fact of research life, coupled with the need for funding in order to pursue a scientific career, produces a huge incentive for investigators both to produce positive results and to publish them. It also encourages researchers to conduct preliminary small studies that are of low quality—that lack, for example, the addition of a double-blinded placebo control group—and so are more likely to produce a negative than a positive finding.

While the dramas behind these scenarios may not appear to amount to very much in individual studies, their cumulative effect can become quite concentrated at the top of the research food chain, where systematic reviews reside. There, small positive trials begin to predominate, are not counterbalanced by equally small but unpublished negative trials, and can easily overwhelm the effect of a larger, high-quality trial in a systematic review. And in the Cochrane CAM reviews that I am about to present, small trials (often published a couple of decades before the CONSORT statement was formulated) are the rule rather than the exception.

But despite the various flies in the ointment of research that I've identified, including some other biases, conscious or unconscious, that are present in all types of trials, the Cochrane systematic reviews remain an amazing empirical tool and are at least designed to produce the most unbiased assessments possible as to whether or not a therapy (conventional or CAM) is effective.

THE COCHRANE CAM SYSTEMATIC REVIEWS

I have attempted to objectively classify the ninety-eight systematic reviews I located as providing either a positive (+) or negative (−)

conclusion regarding the effectiveness of the therapy in question, based upon the reviewers' own assessments. Negative designations included scenarios in which the therapy was judged to be not effective or the evidence was considered to be too scant or of too low a quality to make a determination one way or another. In some cases I didn't think the reviewers' conclusions could be classified either way; hence I designated these as basically equivocal findings ($\approx$).

Because of the number of reviews involved, I don't describe any of them in detail, but instead offer a quick perusal of the evaluated therapies in order to provide a gestalt of the type of evidence available. Also, since interpreting the results of a systematic review has been shown to be an error-prone activity in and of itself, I have attempted to make my positive, negative, and equivocal designations as objective as possible by directly quoting the reviewers' bottom-line judgments from the conclusion section of their abstracts.[10] On rare occasion I have included a quote from the review itself, in which case I have provided in the notes the page number from which it was taken.

1 −

Acupuncture for Acute Stroke

"Acupuncture appeared to be safe but without clear evidence of benefit."[11]

2 −

Acupuncture for Asthma

"There is not enough evidence to make recommendations about the value of acupuncture in asthma treatment."[12]

3 –

Acupuncture for Bell's Palsy

"The quality of the included trials was inadequate to allow any conclusion about the efficacy of acupuncture."[13]

4 ≈

Acupuncture for Headache

"Due to the clinical heterogeneity and the poor methodological quality of the included studies, straightforward recommendations for clinical practice cannot be made." "Overall, the existing evidence supports the value of acupuncture for the treatment of idiopathic headaches. However, the quality and amount of evidence are not fully convincing. There is an urgent need for well-planned, large-scale studies to assess the effectiveness and cost-effectiveness of acupuncture under real-life conditions."[14]

5 –

Acupuncture for Depression

"There is insufficient evidence to determine the efficacy of acupuncture compared to medication, or to wait list control or sham acupuncture, in the management of depression. Scientific study design was poor and the number of people studied was small."[15]

6 –

Acupuncture for Elbow Pain

"No benefit lasting more than 24 hours following treatment has been demonstrated."[16]

7 –

Acupuncture for Epilepsy

"The current evidence does not support acupuncture as a treatment for epilepsy."[17]

8 –

Acupuncture for Treatment of Irritable Bowel Syndrome

"There is no evidence to support the use of acupuncture for the treatment of irritable bowel syndrome."[18]

9 +

Acupuncture for Low Back Pain

"The data do not allow firm conclusions about the effectiveness of acupuncture for acute low-back pain. For chronic low-back pain, acupuncture is more effective for pain relief and functional improvement than no treatment or sham treatment immediately after treatment and in the short-term only."[19]

10 +

Acupuncture for Neck Disorders

"There is moderate evidence that acupuncture relieves pain better than some sham treatments."

The only two positive trials involved a sham acupuncture control, and in the reviewers' words, "both studies are of low quality and positive."[20] The other types of controls included sham TENS and other CAM treatments, which, as we've discussed, aren't adequate for acupuncture trials.

11 −

Acupuncture and Related Interventions for Smoking Cessation

"There is no clear evidence that acupuncture, acupressure, laser therapy or electrostimulation are effective for smoking cessation but methodological problems mean that no firm conclusions can be drawn."[21]

12 −

Acupuncture for Shoulder Pain

"Due to a small number of clinical and methodologically diverse trials, little can be concluded from this review."[22]

13 −

Acupuncture for Schizophrenia

"We found insufficient evidence to recommend the use of acupuncture for people with schizophrenia."[23]

14 −

Acupuncture for Stroke Rehabilitation

"Currently there is no clear evidence on the effects of acupuncture on subacute or chronic stroke."[24]

15 +

Acupuncture-Point Stimulation for Chemotherapy-Induced Nausea or Vomiting

"Electroacupuncture is effective for first day vomiting after chemotherapy, but trials considering modern antivomiting drugs are needed."[25]

The latter is easier said than done, since modern antiemetics are so effective that today it is difficult to do trials such as the ones reported in this review. (I learned this in my position as director of research at a CAM center when we tried to perform a definitive study in this area but could not locate chemotherapy patients whose vomiting was not controlled.) Many of the trials making up this review employed a wristband that provided electrical stimulation, hence making blinding quite difficult.

16 –

Auricular Acupuncture for Cocaine Dependence

"There is currently no evidence that auricular acupuncture is effective for the treatment of cocaine dependence."[26]

17 +

Aromatherapy and Massage for Cancer Symptom Relief (Psychological Well-Being) in Patients with Cancer

"Massage and aromatherapy massage confer short term benefits on psychological wellbeing with the evidence on anxiety supported by limited evidence."[27]

Only two trials employing a placebo control were involved, one for massage and one for non-aromatherapy oil.

18 –

Art Therapy for Mental Illness

"Randomised studies have been proven to be possible in this field. The use of art therapy for serious mental illnesses should continue to be under evaluation as its benefits, or harms, are unclear."[28]

19

Artichoke Leaf Extract for High Cholesterol

"Few data from rigorous clinical trials assessing ALE [artichoke leaf extract] for treating hypercholesterolaemia exist. Beneficial effects are reported, the evidence however is not compelling. The limited data on safety suggest only mild, transient and infrequent adverse events with the short term use of ALE. More rigorous clinical trials assessing larger patient samples over longer intervention periods are needed to establish whether ALE is an effective and safe treatment option for patients with hypercholesterolaemia."[29]

20

Balneotherapy (Spa Therapy) for Arthritis

"Because of the methodological flaws an answer about the efficacy of balneotherapy cannot be provided at this time."[30]

21

Biofeedback and/or Sphincter Exercises for the Treatment of Fecal Incontinence in Adults

"The limited number of identified trials together with their methodological weaknesses do not allow a reliable assessment of the possible role of sphincter exercises and biofeedback therapy in the management of people with faecal incontinence."[31]

22 +

Cernilton (Component Found in Rye-Grass Pollen) for Prostatic Hyperplasia

"The Cernilton trials analyzed were limited by short duration, limited numbers of enrollees, gaps in reported outcomes, and unknown quality of the preparations utilized....The available evidence suggests Cernilton is well tolerated and modestly improves overall urologic symptoms including nocturia."[32]

23 –

Chelation Therapy for Heart Disease

"At present, there is insufficient evidence to decide on the effectiveness or ineffectiveness of chelation therapy in improving clinical outcomes of patients with atherosclerotic cardiovascular disease."[33]

24 –

Iron Chelating Agents for Treating Malaria

"There are insufficient data for any conclusions for both agents tested. There are non-significant trends towards harm (death) and potential benefit (fewer seizures) with DFO [one of the chelating agents]."[34]

25 ≈

Complementary and Alternative Therapies for Pain Management in Labor

"Acupuncture and hypnosis may be beneficial for the management of pain during labor. However, few complementary therapies have been subjected to proper scientific study and the number of women studied is small."[35]

26 –

Complementary and Miscellaneous Interventions for Nocturnal Enuresis in Children

"There was weak evidence to support the use of hypnosis, psychotherapy, acupuncture and chiropractic but it was provided in each case by single small trials, some of dubious methodological rigor."[36]

27 –

Dan Shen (A Type of Traditional Chinese Herb) Agents for Acute Ischemic Stroke

"There were too few patients and outcome events to draw reliable conclusions from the present data. The methodological qualities of all included studies were poor."[37]

28 −

Echinacea for Preventing and Treating the Common Cold

"There is some evidence that preparations based on the aerial parts of *Echinacea purpurea* might be effective for the early treatments of colds in adults but results are not fully consistent."[38]

29 +

Electrical Stimulation for Post-stroke Shoulder Pain

"The evidence from randomized controlled trials so far does not confirm or refute that ES [electrical stimulation] around the shoulder after stroke influences reports of pain, but there do appear to be benefits for passive humeral lateral rotation.... Further studies are required."[39]

This finding was based on only one small trial (twenty participants per group) employing placebo controls. The other two employed non-sham controls.

30 −

Electrotherapy for Neck Disorders

"We can not make any definitive statements on electrotherapy for mechanical neck disorders. The current evidence on Galvanic current (direct or pulsed), iontophoresis, TENS, EMS,

PEMF, and permanent magnets is either lacking, limited, or conflicting."[40]

31 +

Electromagnetic Fields for Osteoarthritis

"Current evidence suggests that electrical stimulation therapy may provide significant improvements for knee OA [osteoarthritis], but further studies are required to confirm whether the statistically significant results shown in these trials confer to important benefits." "In summary, this meta-analysis did not reveal clinically important results, but the analysis was limited by the paucity of literature on electrical stimulation for OA."[41]

32 –

Electromagnetic Therapy for Pressure Sores

"The results suggest no evidence of a benefit in using electromagnetic therapy to treat pressure sores. However the possibility of a beneficial or harmful effect cannot be ruled out due to the fact there were only two trials with methodological limitations and small numbers of patients."[42]

33 –

Electromagnetic Therapy for Treating Venous Leg Ulcers

"There is currently no reliable evidence of benefit of electromagnetic therapy in the healing of venous leg ulcers."[43]

34 −

Feverfew for Preventing Migraine Headaches

"There is insufficient evidence from randomized, double-blind trials to suggest an effect of feverfew over and above placebo for preventing migraine.... The efficacy of feverfew for the prevention of migraine has not been established beyond reasonable doubt."[44]

35 −

Garlic for Preventing Preeclampsia and Its Complications

"There is insufficient evidence to recommend garlic intake for preventing pre-eclampsia and its complications."[45]

36 +

Glucosamine for Osteoarthritis

"This update includes 20 studies with 2570 patients. Pooled results from studies using a non-Rotta preparation [Rotta is a pharmaceutical company] or adequate allocation concealment failed to show benefit in pain and WOMAC [Western Ontario and McMaster Osteoarthritis Index, which is the recommended measure for osteoarthritis research] function while those studies evaluating the Rotta preparation show that glucosamine was superior to placebo in the treatment of pain and function impairment resulting from systematic osteoarthritis. WOMAC outcomes of pain, stiffness and function did not show a superiority of glucosamine over placebo for either Rotta or non-Rotta preparations of glucosamine."[46]

This review was basically made obsolete by the large high-quality RCT published after its completion (trial 4 in Chapter 11). See also the detailed discussion of this review in the case study at the end of this chapter.

37 +

Herbal Therapy for Osteoarthritis

"The evidence for avocado-soybean unsaponifiables in the treatment of osteoarthritis is convincing but evidence for the other herbal interventions is insufficient to either recommend or discourage their use."[47]

38 −

Herbal Therapy for Rheumatoid Arthritis

"There appears to be some potential benefit for the use of GLA [gamma-linolenic acid, an omega-6 fatty acid found in vegetable oil] in rheumatoid arthritis although further studies are required to establish optimum dosage and duration of treatment. The single studies are inconclusive."[48]

39 +

Herbal Therapy for Low Back Pain

"Harpagophytum Procumbens [devil's claw], Salix Alba [white willow bark] and Capsicum Frutescens [hot peppers] seem to reduce pain more than placebo. Additional trials testing these herbal medicines against standard treatments are needed. The quality of reporting in these trials was generally poor."[49]

Perhaps the reason the authors felt that additional studies were needed was that the two placebo-controlled trials evaluating devil's claw were conducted by the same German investigator and one of the two trials evaluating white willow bark was also conducted by this individual. (The remaining study, fortunately, was conducted by a different German investigator.)

40 +

Pygeum africanum *for Benign Prostatic Hyperplasia*

"A standardized preparation of *Pygeum africanum* may be a useful treatment option for men with lower urinary symptoms consistent with benign prostatic hyperplasia. However, the reviewed studies were small in size, were of short duration, used varied doses and preparations and rarely reported outcomes using standardized validated measures of efficacy."[50]

41 –

Herbs for Hepatitis B

"Some Chinese medicinal herbs may work in chronic hepatitis B. However, the evidence is too weak to recommend any single herb. Rigorously designed, randomised, double-blind, placebo-controlled trials are required."[51]

42 –

Medicinal Herbs for Hepatitis C Virus Infection

"There is no firm evidence of efficacy of any medicinal herbs for HCV infection. Medicinal herbs for HCV infection should not be used outside randomized clinical trials."[52]

43 ≈

Herbal Medicines for Viral Myocarditis

"Some herbal medicines may have anti-arrhythmia effects in suspected viral myocarditis. However, interpretation of these findings should be careful due to the low methodological quality, small sample size, and limited number of trials on individual herbs."[53]

Only one of the forty herbal trials included employed an herbal placebo.

44 –

Herbal Medicines for Treating HIV Infection and AIDS

"There is insufficient evidence to support the use of herbal medicines in HIV-infected individuals and AIDS patients."[54]

45 +

Chinese Herbal Medicine for Schizophrenia

"Chinese herbal medicines, given in a Western biomedical context, may be beneficial for people with schizophrenia when combined with anti psychotics." "Overall, the quality of reporting on randomization and blinding was poor, with no studies describing how either randomization and/or blinding was conducted…ensuring participants are blind to their treatment is especially difficult when herbal medicines are given in a liquid form (which they were in these studies) which can be readily seen, smelt, and tasted…this obviously raises questions of the placebo effect on these results."[55]

46 –

Chinese Herbal Medicines for Type 2 Diabetes Mellitus

"We are still waiting for firm evidence on Chinese herbal medicines for treatment of non-insulin-dependent diabetes."[56]

47 –

Chinese Herbs Combined with Western Medicine for SARS

"Chinese herbs combined with Western medicines made no difference in decreasing morbidity versus Western medicines alone. It is possible that Chinese herbs combined with Western medicines may improve symptoms, quality of life, and lung in-filtrate absorption and decrease the corticosteroid dosage for SARS patients. The evidence is weak because of the poor quality of the included trials."[57]

48 −

Chinese Medicinal Herbs for Chemotherapy Side Effects in Colorectal Cancer Patients

"Due to the methodological limitations of the studies, there is no robust demonstration of benefit."[58]

None of the four trials mentioned employing a placebo, and all were published in Chinese CAM journals.

49 −

Chinese Medicinal Herbs for Acute Bronchitis

"There is insufficient quality data to recommend the routine use of Chinese herbs for acute bronchitis. The benefit found in this systematic review could be due to publication bias and study-design limitations of the individual studies."[59]

50 ≈

Chinese Medicinal Herbs for Acute Pancreatitis

"Some Chinese medicinal herbs may work in acute pancreatitis. However the evidence is too weak to recommend any single herb. Rigorously designed, randomized, double-blind, placebo-controlled trials are required."[60]

The authors also noted: "All of these trials were published in Chinese and...none of the articles described the method of randomization."

51 –

Chinese Medicinal Herbs for Influenza

"The evidence in this review was far from conclusive for clinical decision making about traditional Chinese medicinal herbs in the treatment of influenza."[61]

52 ≈

Chinese Herbal Medicine for Atopic Eczema

"Chinese herbal mixtures may be effective in the treatment of atopic eczema. However, only four small poorly reported RCTs of the same product, Zemaphyte, were found and the results were heterogeneous. Further, well-designed, larger scale trials are required, but Zemaphyte is no longer being manufactured."[62]

53 –

Ginkgo biloba *for Acute Ischemic Stroke*

"There was no convincing evidence from trials of sufficient methodological quality to support the routine use of *Ginkgo biloba* extract to promote recovery from stroke."[63]

54 –

Ginkgo biloba *for Cognitive Impairment*

"Many of the early trials used unsatisfactory methods, were small, and we cannot exclude publication bias. Overall there is promising evidence of improvement in cognition and function associated with Ginkgo. However, the three more modern trials [conducted between 1997 and 2000] show inconsistent results. Our view is that there is need for a large trial using modern methodology and permitting an intention-to-treat analysis to provide robust estimates of the size and mechanism of any treatment effects."[64]

55 –

Ginkgo biloba *for Tinnitus*

"The limited evidence did not demonstrate that Ginkgo biloba was effective for tinnitus which is a primary complaint. There was no reliable evidence to address the question of Ginkgo biloba for tinnitus associated with cerebral insufficiency."[65]

56 +

Horse Chestnut Seed Extract for Chronic Venous Insufficiency

"The evidence presented implies that HCSE [horse chestnut seed extract] is an efficacious and safe short-term treatment for chronic venous insufficiency. However, several caveats exist and more rigorous RCTs are required to confirm the efficacy of this treatment option."[66]

Of the seventeen trials that went into this review, fifteen were published in Germany, one in France, and one in Brazil.

57 –

Hypnosis for Schizophrenia

"The studies in this field are few, small, poorly reported and out-dated. Hypnosis could be helpful for people with schizophrenia but to ascertain this requires better designed, conducted and reported randomized studies."[67]

58 –

Hypnotherapy for Smoking Cessation

"We have not shown that hypnotherapy has a greater effect on six month quit rates than other interventions or no treatment. The effects of hypnotherapy on smoking cessation claimed by uncontrolled studies were not confirmed by analysis of random-ized controlled trials."[68]

59 –

Homeopathy for Influenza

"Oscillococcinum [a popular homeopathic remedy based on bacteria supposedly present in the Spanish flu of 1917] probably reduces the duration of illness in patients presenting with influenza symptoms. Though promising, the data are not strong enough to make a general recommendation to use Oscillococcinum for first-line treatment of influenza and influenza-like syndrome. Further research is warranted but required sample sizes are large. Current evidence does not support a preventative effect of homeopathy in influenza and influenza-like syndromes."[69]

60 –

Homeopathy for Induction of Labor

"There is insufficient evidence to recommend the use of caulophyllum [also called blue cohosh] as a method of labour induction. It is likely that the demand for complementary medicine will continue and women will continue to consult a homoeopath during their pregnancy. Although caulophyllum is a commonly used homoeopathic therapy to induce labour, the treatment strategy used in this trial may not reflect routine practice of homoeopathy. It may be more appropriate to undertake further evaluation of individualised homeopathic therapies for induction of labour in future clinical trials."[70]

61 –

Homeopathy for Chronic Asthma

"There is not enough evidence to reliably assess the possible role of homeopathy in asthma....Currently the major obstacle to clinically relevant research is a paucity of information, systematically acquired, on (a) what homeopaths actually do...and (b) how patients respond to homeopathic treatment."[71]

62 –

Intercessory Prayer for Health

"Data in this review are too inconclusive to guide those wishing to uphold or refute the effect of intercessory prayer on health care outcomes. In the light of the best available data, there are no grounds to change current practices. There are few completed trials of the value of intercessory prayer, and the evidence presented so far is interesting enough to justify further study."

"If prayer is seen as a human endeavour it may or may not be beneficial, and further trials could uncover this. It could be the case that any effects are due to elements beyond present scientific understanding that will, in time, be understood. If any benefit derives from God's response to prayer it may be beyond any such trials to prove or disprove."[72]

63 +

Kava for Anxiety

"Compared with placebo, kava extract appears to be an effective symptomatic treatment option for anxiety. The effect lacks robustness and is based on a relatively small sample."[73]

64 –

Laetrile Treatment for Cancer

"The claim that Laetrile has beneficial effects for cancer patients is not supported by data from controlled clinical trials."[74]

65 −

Low-Level Laser Therapy for Osteoarthritis

"For osteoarthritis, the results are conflicting in different studies.... The pooled results indicated no effect of one month of low level laser therapy on pain or overall patient-rated assessment of disease activity."[75]

66 +

Low-Level Laser Therapy for Rheumatoid Arthritis

"LLLT [low-level laser therapy] could be considered for short-term treatment for relief of pain and morning stiffness for RA [rheumatoid arthritis] patients, particularly since it has few side-effects."[76]

67 ≈

Massage for Back Pain

"Massage might be beneficial for patients with subacute and chronic non-specific low-back pain, especially when combined with exercises and education. The evidence suggests that acupuncture massage is more effective than classic massage, but this needs confirmation."[77]

I downgraded this review from a guarded positive rating to equivocal because it employed studies contrasting massage to *other* CAM and active therapies. In the reviewer's words: "Massage was inferior to manipulation and TENS; massage was equal to corsets and exercises; and massage was superior to relaxation therapy, acupuncture and self-care education." In this chapter we are really not interested in whether one CAM therapy is better or worse than another, since all this may mean is that one type of placebo is more effective than another.

68 –

Massage and Touch for Dementia

"Massage and touch may serve as alternatives or complements to other therapies for the management of behavioral, emotional and perhaps other conditions associated with dementia. More research is needed, however, to provide definitive evidence about the benefits of these interventions."[78]

69 –

Massage for Mechanical Neck Disorders

"No recommendations for practice can be made at this time because the effectiveness of massage for neck pain remains uncertain."[79]

70 –

Meditation Therapy for Anxiety Disorders

"The small number of studies included in this review do not permit any conclusions to be drawn on the effectiveness of meditation therapy for anxiety disorders."[80]

71 –

S-*adenosyl-L-methionine (SAMe) for Alcoholic Liver Diseases*

"This systematic review could not demonstrate any significant effect of SAMe on mortality, liver related mortality, mortality or liver transplantation, and liver complications of patients with alcoholic liver disease. SAMe should not be used for alcoholic liver disease outside randomized clinical trials."[81]

72 –

Speleotherapy for Asthma

"The available evidence does not permit a reliable conclusion as to whether speleo-therapeutic interventions [a process that involves using the health-enhancing effect of salt mines or caves] are effective for the treatment of chronic asthma. Randomized controlled trials with long-term follow-up are necessary."[82]

73 –

Spinal Manipulative Therapy for Low Back Pain

"There is no evidence that spinal manipulative therapy is superior to other standard treatments for patients with acute or chronic low-back pain."[83]

74 −

Spinal Manipulative Therapy for Primary and Secondary Dysmenorrhea

"Overall there is no evidence to suggest that spinal manipulation is effective in the treatment of primary and secondary dysmenorrhoea."[84]

75 ≈

Noninvasive Physical Treatments (e.g., Spinal Manipulation, Cranial Electrotherapy) for Chronic, Recurrent Headache

"A few non-invasive physical treatments may be effective as prophylactic treatments for chronic/recurrent headaches."

"The evidence for efficacy or inefficacy of the different non-invasive physical treatments for the various types of headaches rests on separate trials."

Of the twenty-two trials included, eighteen did not employ a credible placebo group, and two of the remaining four scored only a 1 on the 5-point Jadad scale.[85]

76 −

Manual Therapies for Asthma

"There is insufficient evidence to support the use of manual therapies for patients with asthma. There is a need to conduct adequately-sized RCTs that examine the effects of manual therapies on clinically relevant outcomes. Future trials should maintain observer blinding for outcome assessments, and report on the costs of care and adverse events. Currently, there is insufficient evidence to support or refute the use of manual therapy for patients with asthma."[86]

77 –

Milk Thistle for Alcoholic and Hepatitis Liver Diseases

"Our results question the beneficial effects of milk thistle for patients with alcoholic and/or hepatitis B or C virus liver diseases and highlight the lack of high-quality evidence to support this intervention."[87]

78 –

Music Therapy for People with Dementia

"The methodological quality and the reporting of the included studies were too poor to draw any useful conclusions."[88]

79 +

Music Therapy for Schizophrenia or Schizophrenia-like Illnesses

"Music therapy as an addition to standard care helps people with schizophrenia to improve their global state and may also improve mental state and functioning if a sufficient number of music therapy sessions are provided."[89]

None of the studies employed a placebo control.

80 ≈

Prolotherapy Injections (Repeated Injection of Irritating Solutions) for Chronic Low Back Pain

"There is conflicting evidence regarding the efficacy of prolotherapy injections in reducing pain and disability in patients with chronic low-back pain. Conclusions are confounded by...the presence of co-interventions. There was no evidence that prolotherapy injections alone were more effective than control injections alone."[90]

81 +

St. John's Wort for Depression

"Available evidence suggests that several specific extracts of St. John's wort may be effective for treating mild to moderate depression, although the data are not fully convincing."[91]

Only two of the review's twenty-six trials comparing St. John's wort to placebo were conducted in the United States, and both were negative (see the high-quality *JAMA* articles presented in Chapter 11, trials 5 and 6).

82 +

Serenoa repens *for Benign Prostatic Hyperplasia*

"*Serenoa repens,* a herbal medicine, provides mild to moderate improvement in urinary symptoms and flow measures for men with enlarged prostate glands (benign prostatic hyperplasia)."[92]

This 2002 review is trumped by the high-quality negative RCT on saw palmetto published in 2006 in NEJM (Chapter 11, trial 13).

83 –

Tai Chi for Treating Rheumatoid Arthritis

"Tai Chi based exercise programs had no clinically important or statistically significant effect on most outcomes of disease activity, which included activities of daily living, tender and swollen joints and patient global overall rating. For range of motion, Tai Chi participants had statistically significant and clinically important improvements in ankle plantar flexion."[93]

The improvement in ankle plantar flexion was based on one small poor-quality trial that compared tai chi to no treatment at all.

84 –

Ultrasound for Ankle Sprains

"The extent and quality of the available evidence for the effects of ultrasound therapy for acute ankle sprains is limited. The results of four placebo-controlled trials do not support the use of ultrasound in the treatment of ankle sprains."[94]

85 –

Ultrasound for Pressure Sores

"The results suggest no apparent evidence of a benefit of ultrasound therapy in the treatment of pressure sores. However the possibility of a beneficial or a harmful effect cannot be ruled out due to the small number of trials with methodological limitations and small numbers of participants."[95]

86 –

Ultrasound for Osteoarthritis

"Ultrasound therapy appears to have no benefit over placebo or short wave diathermy for people with hip or knee OA. These conclusions are limited by the poor reporting of the characteristics of the device, the population, the stage of OA, therapeutic application of the ultrasound and overall low methodological quality of the trials included. No conclusions can be drawn about the use of ultrasound in smaller joints such as the wrist or hands."[96]

87 –

Therapeutic Ultrasound for Postpartum Perineal Pain and Dyspareunia

"There is not enough evidence to evaluate the use of ultrasound in treating perineal pain and/or dyspareunia following childbirth."[97]

88 ≈

Ultrasound for Rheumatoid Arthritis

"The reviewers concluded that ultrasound in combination with exercises, faradic current and wax bath treatment modalities is not supported and cannot be recommended. Ultrasound alone can, however, be used on the hand to increase grip strength, and to a lesser extent and based on borderline results, increase wrist dorsal flexion, decrease morning stiffness, reduce the number of swollen joints, and reduce the number of painful joints. It is important to note that these conclusions are limited by methodological considerations such as poor quality of the included trials, the low number of clinical trials, and the small number of study participants."[98]

Actually, both conclusions, the negative one and the positive one, were based upon only one trial each. I probably shouldn't have included the review, but technically it consisted of multiple trials—just not multiple trials addressing the same outcome.

89 +

Therapeutic Ultrasound for Venous Leg Ulcers

"The available evidence does suggest a possible benefit of ultrasound therapy in the healing of venous leg ulcers, however, only seven small studies were identified, and this conclusion needs interpreting."

"Overall the methodological quality of the studies included in this review was poor."[99]

Of the seven studies, three were RCTs employing a sham control, only one of which (with a grand total of thirteen participants per group) achieved statistical significance.

90 –

Transcranial Magnetic Stimulation for Obsessive-Compulsive Disorder

"There are currently insufficient data from randomised controlled trials to draw any conclusions about the efficacy of transcranial magnetic stimulation in the treatment of obsessive-compulsive disorder."[100]

91 –

Transcranial Magnetic Stimulation for Depression

"The information in this review suggests that there is no strong evidence for benefit from using transcranial magnetic stimulation to treat depression, although the small sample sizes do not exclude the possibility of benefit."[101]

92 +

TENS for Osteoarthritis

"TENS and AL-TENS are shown to be effective in pain control over placebo in this review. Heterogeneity of the included studies was observed, which might be due to the different study designs and outcomes used. More well designed studies with a standardized protocol and adequate numbers of participants are needed to conclude the effectiveness of TENS in the treatment of OA of the knee."[102]

93 –

TENS for Low Back Pain

"There is limited and inconsistent evidence to support the use of TENS as an isolated intervention in the management of chronic lower back pain.... The available evidence supporting the use of TENS as an isolated treatment modality is limited and conflicting."[103]

94 –

TENS for Chronic Pain

"The results of this review are inconclusive; the published trials do not provide information on the stimulation parameters which are most likely to provide optimum pain relief, nor do they answer questions about long-term effectiveness. Large multi-centre randomised controlled trials of TENS in chronic pain are urgently needed."[104]

95 –

TENS for Dementia

"Although a number of studies suggest that TENS may produce short lived improvements in some neuropsychological or behavioural aspects of dementia, the limited presentation and availability of data from these studies does not allow definite conclusions on the possible benefits of this intervention. Since most of the currently published studies are well designed, although the numbers of subjects in each study is small, analysis of the complete original data from these and/or future studies may allow more definitive conclusions to be drawn."[105]

96 ≈

TENS for Rheumatoid Arthritis in the Hand

"There are conflicting effects of TENS on pain outcomes in patients with RA. AL-TENS [acupuncture-like TENS] is beneficial for reducing pain intensity and improving muscle power scores over placebo while, conversely, C-TENS [conventional TENS] resulted in no clinical benefit on pain intensity compared with placebo. However, C-TENS resulted in a clinical benefit on patient assessment of change in disease over AL-TENS. More well designed studies with a standardized protocol and adequate number of subjects are needed to fully conclude the effect of C-TENS and AL-TENS in the treatment of RA of the hand."[106]

97 +

TENS for Dysmenorrhea

"High frequency TENS was found to be effective for the treatment of dysmenorrhoea by a number of small trials. The minor adverse effects reported in one trial requires further investigation. There is insufficient evidence to determine the effectiveness of low frequency TENS in reducing dysmenorrhoea."[107]

98 –

Therapeutic Touch for Healing Acute Wounds

"There is insufficient evidence that TT [therapeutic touch] promotes healing of acute wounds."[108]

SO WHAT DOES IT ALL MEAN?

Well, in the first place, these results as analyzed in *relatively* high-quality systematic reviews are certainly more positive than the findings of individual trials published in the high-quality medical journals that we examined in Chapter 11. They are a good deal less than overwhelming, however, since I counted twenty-one out of the ninety-eight reviews (or roughly 21 percent) as providing positive conclusions. And even that small number is a little deceptive, because quite a few of the positive reviews cannot be taken at face value. Table 12.1 presents the twenty-one positive reviews along with some of the reasons for interpretative caution. (Note that some of these reviews could have been listed under more than one column; I have simply chosen the weakness I considered most problematic for a particular review.)

In hindsight, I shouldn't have included two of the reviews (number 29, on electrical stimulation for shoulder pain, and number 79, on music therapy) because one involved only one small placebo-controlled trial and the other involved none. And as we've discussed, two more reviews (number 36, on glucosamine, and number 82, on *Serenoa repens,* or saw palmetto) were trumped by negative high-quality, placebo-controlled trials after the reviews in question were completed. This brings our overall portion of positive reviews down to 17 percent, which—compared to the only benchmark that I'm aware is available to date—is far below the 85 percent rate of positive reviews found in a larger survey of systematic reviews assessing the effectiveness of educational and behavioral (including a good number of health) interventions.[110] I think

Table 12.1. Positive Cochrane Systematic Reviews

Review Number and Subject	≤1 Placebo Control Group	Trumped by Later Large, High-Quality RCT	No English-Speaking Confirmation of Positive Results	Therapies with Suspect Placebos or That Employ Single Blinding
9: Acupuncture for low back pain			√	
10: Acupuncture for neck disorders				
15: Acupuncture/ acupressure for vomiting				
17: Aromatherapy for cancer symptoms				
22: Cernilton for prostatic hyperplasia			√	
29: Electrical stimulation for shoulder pain	√			
31: Electromagnetic fields for osteoarthritis				√
36: Glucosamine for osteoarthritis		√		
37: Herbal therapy for osteoarthritis			√	
39: Herbal therapy for low back pain			√	
40: *Pygeum africanum* for swollen prostrate			√	

(*continued*)

Table 12.1. (*continued*)

Review Number and Subject	≤1 Placebo Control Group	Trumped by Later Large, High-Quality RCT	No English-Speaking Confirmation of Positive Results	Therapies with Suspect Placebos or That Employ Single Blinding
45: Chinese herbs for schizophrenia				√
56: Horse chestnut extract for venous insufficiency			√	
63: Kava for anxiety			√	
66: Laser therapy for rheumatoid arthritis				
79: Music therapy for schizophrenia	√			
81: St. John's wort for depression			√	
82: *Serenoa repens* for swollen prostate		√		
89: Ultrasound for venous leg ulcers				
92: TENS for osteoarthritis				√
97: TENS for menstrual cramps				√
Percentage of positive reviews with each weakness	19%	17%	9%	5%

there is no question that publication bias, small-study effects, and all the other myriad sources of research bias we've discussed previously could easily account for most of such a figure, but let's disregard those factors for a moment and turn to more flaws that the biostatistical obsessive-compulsive in me can't avoid bringing up. If we further knock out reviews that did not include positive confirmation from a study conducted in an English-speaking country, the 17 percent positive rate declines to 9 percent. Eliminating reviews involving suspect controls, the positive rate drops to 5 percent—which, I don't believe that I have to mention (but of course will anyway), is exactly the same as Sir Ronald Fisher's figure.

NON-COCHRANE REVIEWS: AN EXAMPLE

The truth is, though, that Cochrane reviews are not representative of CAM systematic reviews in general. There is an entire realm of non-Cochrane-based CAM reviews that I haven't yet discussed because their assessments are questionable in light of the following circumstances: such reviews are more likely to be conducted by CAM proponents, less critical (and less cognizant) of the abysmal methodological quality that tends to characterize CAM trials, and less hesitant to base their bottom-line conclusions on poorly controlled research coming from tiny, specialized CAM publications that serve as little more than mouthpieces for the particular therapies they represent.

I would like to illustrate my concerns with non-Cochrane reviews via the best-known and probably most frequently cited positive CAM meta-analysis yet conducted. I find this one particularly interesting for three reasons. First, from a technical perspective, it is an extremely well done systematic review and was published in a credible medical journal. Second, unlike so many CAM treatments, it involves a genre of therapy for which credible placebos can be constructed even more easily than is the case for conventional drugs (since this therapy's medications have neither taste nor smell). Third, as will be discussed in the next chapter, it is a therapy for which absolutely no scientifically defensible biochemical mechanism of action has been proposed (and for which there is probably more skepticism among modern physicians and scientists than just about any other CAM therapy). The therapy, of course, is homeopathy.

Are the Clinical Effects of Homeopathy Placebo Effects? A Meta-analysis of Placebo-Controlled Trials

K. Linde, N. Clausius, G. Ramirez, D. Melchart, F. Eitel, L. V. Hedges, and W. B. Jonas

This review of homeopathic research begins with an understatement of the obvious: "Homeopathy seems scientifically implausible, but has widespread use. We aimed to assess whether the clinical effect reported in randomized controlled trials of homeopathic remedies is equivalent to that reported for placebo."[111] After what appeared to be a very thorough and systematic search of the literature, the authors located eighty-nine usable trials published between 1943 and 1995 containing a median of sixty patients per study. The trials came from thirteen different countries and were written in four different languages. Following a through analysis of the studies, a section of which was overseen at least in part by coauthor Larry Hedges, one of the most widely respected meta-analytic statisticians, the authors mildly but definitively concluded: "The results of our meta-analysis are not compatible with the hypothesis that the clinical effects of homeopathy are completely due to placebo." They did, however, add a fairly important qualifier in their very next sentence: "But there is insufficient evidence from these studies that any single type of homoeopathic treatment is clearly effective in any one clinical condition."[112]

This second sentence is really a big disclaimer, but still, looking at the totality of the evidence, the authors did find that in general patients receiving homeopathic remedies fared better than their randomly assigned counterparts who received placebos. So should we conclude that homeopathy is effective? Let's allow some other people to have their say before I answer this one.

The review attracted so much interest that Edzard Ernst, who himself had conducted one of the homeopathic trials included in the Linde meta-analysis, performed what he aptly titled (no, I'm not making this up) "A Systematic Review of Systematic Reviews of Homeopathy." Therein he reported finding seventeen such reviews, six of which were reanalyses of the original work by Linde and colleagues just discussed. (This isn't as uncommon in academia as you might think; Gene Glass's psychotherapy meta-analysis spawned several dozen others, but unlike the homeopathy reanalyses they generally confirmed his original finding.) Of the eleven independent homeopathy systematic reviews, *only two could be construed as positive*. Ernst's overall conclusion regarding these eleven reviews was: "Collectively they failed to provide strong evidence in favor of homeopathy. In particular, there was no condition which responds convincingly better to homeopathic treatment than to placebo" and "No homeopathic remedy was demonstrated to yield clinical evidence that [is] convincingly different from placebo. It is concluded that the best clinical evidence for homeopathy available to date does not warrant positive recommendations for use in clinical practice."[113]

Still, to be fair, two of these eleven reviews could be construed as basically positive (and 2 divided by 11 equals 18 percent, which is very close to the unadjusted figure we obtained from the Cochrane reviews). It is interesting, however, that one of these two positive reviews also reported that the only multisite clinical trial conducted in this area was definitively negative.[114] As mentioned previously, multicenter trials are one way of simulating that most cherished stamp of scientific credibility, independent replication. It's not a great sign, then, that this rare CAM example of a multisite trial produced a definitively negative result (the only other one we've discussed in any detail were the acupuncture and dental surgery trials presented in Chapter 8, which also happened to be negative).

And on a related note, what about the aforementioned six re-analyses of the larger systematic review by Linde and colleagues? These are, after all, another form of replication. Basically, in those reanalyses that considered only the *highest*-quality trials, the highly touted positive effect for homeopathy disappeared.[115] Personally, I find this as telling as the negative multicenter homeopathic trial result, especially since two of these reanalyses were conducted by Klaus Linde, the original author of the meta-analysis in question.

So if everyone else can do a reanalysis of this study based upon a reconsideration of the quality of research, why not your author? Clearly, I have a strong antipathy toward poor-quality research in general, but I'll base my reanalysis in part upon a facet of quality that is relatively unique to CAM. This involves CAM research published in *therapy-specific* CAM journals, which are more prone to publish positive results that reflect well on their specialties (whether acupuncture, traditional Chinese medicine, or homeopathy) than they are to publish negative ones—a practice that may well be innocent and simply subsumed under the category of unconscious publication bias. With that said, note the following journal sources of the vast majority of the trials that Klaus Linde and colleagues cited in their original, positive meta-analysis; many of these sources contributed multiple trials, and one of them actually contributed fourteen.

> *Homéopathie*
> *Berlin Journal on Research in Homeopathy*
> *British Homeopathic Journal*
> *British Homeopathic Research Group Communications*
> *Journal of the American Institute of Homeopathy*
> *Homéopathie Française*
> *Revue Homeopatia*
> *Allgemeine Homoopathische Zeitung*
> *Homint R&D Newsletter*
> *Midlands Homoeopathy Research Group*

This is probably one of those times that I should press the personal bias buzzer, so allow me to cite the following simple fact: 98 percent of the eighty-nine homeopathic trials cited by Linde and colleagues were published in non-U.S. and/or homeopathic journals or were listed as student theses in foreign universities. Only two trials (2 percent) came from American scientific journals (*Archives of Emergency Medicine* and *Pediatrics*).

And that is all there is to my reanalysis, the conclusion of which is consonant with yet another reanalysis completed by Ernst in which he concluded that taking the quality of these homeopathic trials into account produced a bottom-line conclusion that "can be seen as the ultimate epidemiological proof that homeopathic remedies are, in fact, placebos."[116]

REANALYSIS OF THE MOST POSITIVE CAM COCHRANE REVIEW: GLUCOSAMINE FOR ARTHRITIS

Even if Cochrane reviews are the most objective of systematic reviews and seldom conducted by rabid CAM proponents, why shouldn't they be reanalyzed occasionally as well?

The answer is that they should be and they are. One of the beauties of the Cochrane system is that the authors of each review agree to periodically update their systematic reviews as new RCTs become available (and reviews are even withdrawn occasionally when this does not occur). So let's take what may have been the most positive of the CAM Cochrane reviews described in this chapter and see what happened when it was recently reanalyzed.

There is little question that the most positive and most influential of the Cochrane reviews several years ago was number 36, which investigated the effectiveness of glucosamine for treating osteoarthritis. In 1999, the reviewers found thirteen placebo-controlled trials. Their assessment was: "In the 13 RCTs in which glucosamine was compared to placebo, glucosamine was found to be superior in all RCTs, except one."

While this is a strong statement, the reviewers did add an interesting caveat in the second paragraph of their discussion section: "The study by Houpt et al. (1999) deserves further mention since...it is the only North American RCT [and]...unlike the other RCTs, this study failed to show a dramatic efficacy for glucosamine over placebo."[117]

This conclusion and quote came from the first iteration of the glucosamine review, which was conducted in 1999, and the North American RCT they referred to happened to be the most recent trial that the authors reviewed. The systematic review was updated six years later (at the end of 2005) by the same group of authors because several new trials had become available during that time interval. Based upon the addition of these new trials, the reviewers produced a somewhat milder but still positive endorsement of glucosamine:

> This update includes 20 studies with 2570 patients. Pooled results from studies using a non-Rotta preparation or adequate allocation concealment failed to show benefit in pain and WOMAC function while those studies evaluating the Rotta preparation show that glucosamine was superior to placebo in the treatment of pain and function impairment resulting from systematic osteoarthritis. WOMAC outcomes of pain, stiffness and function did not show a superiority of glucosamine over placebo for either Rotta or non-Rotta preparations of glucosamine.[118]

What the reviewers didn't mention was that this wondrous Rotta preparation happened to be investigated primarily by older trials in non-English-speaking countries. The reviewers also didn't mention that among the eight new trials were four reasonably sized studies that were performed in English-speaking countries. Two of these employed more than fifty participants per group (which meets our size criterion used in the last chapter).[119] The other two employed thirty-eight and forty-nine participants per group, respectively (which, while admittedly less than optimal, would certainly not be considered tiny trials).[120] Bottom line? All four were negative.

Study 1: performed in the United States and published in 2004 (93 participants per group). Its conclusion: "Our results suggest that although glucosamine appears to be safe, it is no more effective than placebo in treating the symptoms of knee osteoarthritis."[121]

Study 2: performed in Canada and published in 2004 (68 participants per group). Its conclusion: "In patients with knee OA with at least moderate subjective improvement with prior glucosamine use, this study provides no evidence of symptomatic benefit from continued use of glucosamine sulfate."[122] This study had an unusual design in the sense that only patients who were currently using glucosamine and thought that they were being helped by it were recruited and randomly assigned to either continue to use glucosamine or a placebo.

Study 3: performed in the United Kingdom and published in 2002 (38 participants per group). Its conclusion: "As a symptom modifier in OA patients with a wide range of pain severities, glucosamine sulphate was no more effective than placebo."[123]

Study 4: performed in the United States and published in 2000 (49 participants per group). Its conclusion: "Glucosamine was no better than placebo in reducing pain from osteoarthritis of the knee in this group of patients."[124]

But from my perspective, the nail in this coffin was supplied by an *NEJM* article published on February 23, 2006 (just after this review was updated). Its investigators randomly assigned 1,583 participants to one of five different groups: (1) placebo, (2) glucosamine only, (3) chondroitin only, (4) glucosamine plus chondroitin, and (5) celecoxib (an arthritis medication). As you would expect by now, the results were negative, leading its authors to conclude: "Glucosamine and chondroitin sulfate alone or in combination did not reduce pain effectively in the overall group of patients with osteoarthritis of the knee."[125]

But for the more sadistic among you, those who'd like yet another nail in this particular coffin, I offer a systematic review published in the *Annals of Internal Medicine*. Reviewing twenty trials involving 3,846 patients, the authors concluded: "Large-scale, methodologically sound trials indicate that the symptomatic benefit of chondroitin is minimal or non-existent. Use of chondroitin in routine clinical practice should therefore be discouraged."[126]

And what is your revered author's conclusion? I'll rely on no less an expert than Bob Dylan to provide it for me: "You don't need a weatherman to know which way the wind blows."

So is there sufficient evidence to conclude that *any* CAM therapies are more effective than a placebo? Based upon the evidence presented in both the previous chapter and this one, the bottom-line answer is no. And this conclusion will now be elevated to the status of the book's third principle:

Principle 3: There is no compelling, credible scientific evidence to suggest that any CAM therapy benefits any medical condition or reduces any medical symptom (pain or otherwise) better than a placebo.

CHAPTER THIRTEEN

How CAM Therapies Are Hypothesized to Work

We've now answered three of our four original questions by establishing that (1) there is credible research supporting the existence of a placebo effect for pain, (2) there are plausible biochemical reasons we should believe this research, and (3) there is no credible research to support the existence of any CAM therapeutic effect over and above what can be attributed to the placebo effect. So this brings us to our final task, which is to determine if there is some plausible biochemical reason for us to assume that there *should* be such an effect. Remember, scientists can be wrong, and even the most well-designed placebo-controlled RCTs can sometimes produce false negative results for therapies that in fact do work.

Unfortunately, there is practically no plausible evidence supporting any biochemical mechanisms for CAM therapies. What we'll have to do, therefore, is to concentrate upon the *hypothesized* biological mechanisms of action proposed for CAM therapeutic effects by their proponents.

EVALUATING THE PLAUSIBILITY OF CAM BIOCHEMICAL MECHANISMS OF ACTION

Fortunately, we don't have to evaluate these hypothesized mechanisms of action in a vacuum. We can contrast their plausibility with the physiological and psychological explanations advanced for how placebos work—that is, if I have been successful in supporting the following premise:

If a completely inactive pill, ointment, or procedure (in other words, a placebo), accompanied by the expectation of effectiveness, can result in pain relief, then surely any therapy—no matter how bizarre—that we consider credible enough to seek out (and pay for) can also result in pain relief, compliments of the placebo effect.

In other words, based upon the evidence presented in Chapter 9, we would expect *any* established CAM therapy to be capable of eliciting an analgesic effect, since the main ingredient necessary for such an effect is the belief (or expectation) that a given therapy can provide a therapeutic benefit.[1]

Our task in this chapter, therefore, is to weigh the explanations, theories, or hypotheses advanced for the effectiveness of CAM therapies against those advanced for the placebo effect (not to mention the inferential artifacts that we know are capable of masquerading as therapeutic effects). Of course, if we had uncovered any credible evidence that CAM therapies could cure anything or that they could relieve symptoms better than placebos or placebo-like effects, then this task would have been simpler because we could have evaluated their plausibility on their own merit rather than compare them to something else. Since there is no such evidence, however, we are going to have to wind up relying upon William of Occam's advice after all.

And how does William's principle apply here? Well, given that we know that CAM therapies can be as effective as a placebo, one way to evaluate a CAM therapy's mechanism of action would be to contrast it with the placebo effect's mechanism of action via his parsimony principle. And one way to do *that* would be to simply count up the number of unproven assumptions required by the two competing explanations (that is, for the CAM therapy versus the placebo) to see which involves the fewest assumptions.

In other words, if the CAM therapy du jour requires us to assume the existence of an as-yet-undocumented biological system or unmeasured physical force, then the placebo effect would start out ahead. As discussed in Chapter 10, the placebo effect invokes only a well-documented chemical (endogenous opioids) emanating from a well-documented biological system (the central nervous system) traveling through a well-established physiological route (the bloodstream). Alas, no one anywhere at any time has ever documented the existence of, say, meridians or qi.

I don't expect anyone to be obsessive enough to take out pencil and paper and begin tabulating assumptions. Only a statistician or an accountant would engage in such behavior. Instead, it should suffice to simply keep in mind the gestalt of evidence presented up to this point and then to compare this evidence to the hypothesized mechanisms of action that follow. Or we could use what I like to call Barker of Maryland's ridiculousness test, which allows an evaluator to apply a personal screen to summarily throw out a theory that sounds patently ridiculous. I leave it up to you to apply whichever test—William's or mine—works for you in evaluating these proposed mechanisms.

SELECTED CAM THERAPIES

As was the case in our overview of CAM therapies in Chapter 1, given the truly astounding number of individual CAM therapies currently being practiced, we will by necessity have to be selective in choosing which ones to consider. What I will attempt to do, then, is to make sure that I cover the hypothesized mechanisms of action of some of the more popular modalities, as defined by the surveys discussed in Chapter 1, and those that have been subjected to enough scientific scrutiny to qualify for inclusion in Chapters 11 and 12.

Indigenous Medical Systems

While clinical trials assessing the effectiveness of a few of the individual therapies (such as acupuncture or massage) making up these systems have been conducted, it is extremely difficult to evaluate entire medical systems; hence number-driven evidence for or against these meta-approaches does not exist. In addition, their proposed mechanisms of action are so far removed from modern physiology that no serious scientist would even attempt to study them.

Still, some have medical colleges and schools devoted to training new practitioners (both in their countries of origin and in the West), and someone is paying tuition to attend them. Some even have credentialing examinations, and all have serious, dedicated proponents. Thus we have little choice other than to at least try to see how their individual therapies measure up to the placebo—which is of equally ancient lineage.

Traditional Chinese Medicine

In fairness, we shouldn't forget that TCM's philosophical-physiological system was developed thousands of years ago, when knowledge of human anatomy was extremely rudimentary and no one in any culture had any idea what the function of the various organs and physiological systems were. No one at this time even knew what function blood served. It is also fair, however, not to forget that TCM is being practiced *now* and that no one in the twentieth or twenty-first century has ever measured either qi or the meridians along which it is believed to travel, so it is probably safe to assume that their discovery is not imminent. Yet these unobservable pathways along which this unobservable energy source travels still largely determine the location and method by which needles are placed in the body by modern acupuncturists.

The complex diagnostic system in which a traditional practitioner determines exactly what is out of balance and what is not (by basically "feeling" or assessing unmeasurable pulses or subjectively examining the patient's tongue) should also be fair game, since the results of these examinations are often used to prescribe combinations of therapies, each of which is proposed to have a different therapeutic function but which is no more effective than a placebo. (In a rare fit of compassion, I didn't mention in Chapter 8 the research my center performed in which three experienced TCM physicians examined the same group of rheumatoid arthritis patients and prescribed what they considered to be appropriate therapies. Even though the TCM physicians knew that all of the patients had rheumatoid arthritis, there was no consistency with respect to their diagnoses or their treatment recommendations. In other words, even if this strange, complex, and archaic diagnostic procedure had some physiological basis, it would be worthless, since these experienced practitioners came up with completely different conclusions when examining the same patients.)[2]

That said, therapies such as acupuncture have been adapted and changed over time, even employing electricity-delivering machines (TENS and PENS). Hence some of their practitioners have adopted more physiologically based hypotheses for the mechanism of action of this therapy. Not coincidentally, the most popular of these biochemical explanations (adopted by both TENS and electro-acupuncture) hypothesizes that the electrical stimulation releases endogenous opioids in the brain, which in turn results in pain relief. And indeed, there is some research evidence that some temporary pain relief occurs in both humans and animals in the same manner.[3] Unfortunately, since this happens to be identical to the better documented mechanism for the placebo effect, its evaluation is better transferred from Occam's razor to the even earlier scientific precept to which I've referred:

If it walks like a duck and quacks like a duck, then it's probably a duck (or at least a placebo effect).

Ayurvedic Medicine

While the evaluation of the philosophical basis of ayurvedic medicine is no more a province of science than is a consideration of the merits of Buddhism, nothing remotely similar to the energies *vata*, *pitta*, and *kasha* has ever been documented in biology. And, outside of the use of leeches by certain German scientists mentioned in Chapter 11, bloodletting has fallen from favor as a medical strategy.

Tibetan Medicine

The unique mechanisms of action posited in Tibetan medicine—*chi, schara,* and *badahan*—have failed to be documented by any credible scientists. Indeed, few such scientists are working at a fever pitch to do so.

Nonindigenous Medical Systems

Osteopathic Medicine

To this profession's credit, its malleable philosophical approach (as witnessed by its practitioners' willingness to prescribe pharmaceuticals such as antibiotics in conjunction with other CAM therapy) sets it aside from many of its CAM competitors in the sense that a patient with a real, physiologically based illness could go to his or her osteopath and actually be *cured* (assuming that science has indeed developed a cure for the illness in question). Of course, any CAM therapy could claim the same distinction if its practitioners combined their offerings with, say, tetracycline, but most have too much pride to resort to such practices— and, more to the point, most are not licensed to do so.

On the other hand, there is no evidence for the effectiveness of therapies such as cranial manipulation, nor is there any firm rationale for why the body's natural healing processes need to be "gently prodded," which is one of the rationales for the osteopathic approach to medicine.[4] Fortunately, antibiotics and other pharmaceuticals don't know who prescribes them, an M.D. or a D.O., so it would certainly be inaccurate to say that no firm biochemical mechanism of action exists for *any* component of osteopathic practice.

Naturopathic Medicine

Like osteopaths, naturopaths do have one thing going for them: since they stress a preventive lifestyle consonant with (although more elaborate than) the recommendations of most present-day medical physicians and prefer "natural" substitutes to the pharmaceuticals upon which conventional medicine is based, their prescriptions undoubtedly have fewer side effects than those of most conventional physicians. This means they may be physiologically preferable for one extremely large group of patients: the worried well.

Homeopathy

There is no known physiological principle that can explain why "similars" or "like cures like" should work, nor any chemophysical demonstration of why "succussion" (which, it will be remembered, is a fancy term for vigorous shaking of a medicine) should work, nor any known standardized test among the hundreds on the market to assess water's "memory." Also, nothing else in nature that we know of becomes more potent as it is diluted. So the mechanism of action for this therapy is simply beyond the province of science, since the perfect homeopathic drug has no measurable active ingredient—which could also serve as a very nice definition of a placebo. This is not to say, however, that the evaluation of these drugs' clinical effectiveness is outside the ken of science, since also by definition they are especially suitable for placebo-controlled trials.

In their defense, homeopaths place much more emphasis upon developing a positive, caring relationship with their patients than do most conventional practitioners, and they probably spend more time with them as well, trying to understand both the patient and the genesis of his or her illness. Naturally, this does nothing to dilute (pun intended) the resultant placebo effect that would be expected to accompany the practitioners' assurances that their homeopathic prescriptions were developed specifically for the symptoms that gave rise to the patient's visit in the first place.

Some Individual Therapies

As I've mentioned, there are so many CAM therapies, most of which have been subjected to absolutely no scientific study at all, that I have had to be selective in what I have chosen to discuss in this chapter. The hypothesized mechanisms of action of even the limited sample that follows, however, can be categorized in several different ways. Some posit the presence of mysterious energies that as yet have not been measured by conventional scientific instrumentation. Some posit the existence of as-yet-unobserved physiological systems, while others begin with conventional biological systems and simply extend the principles surrounding their operation far beyond anything yet observed in science. All have one core biological commonality: they all rely upon physiological processes that, as yet, have no biochemically verified basis.

Yoga

Briefly discussed earlier with respect to its probable origins in India, this combination of stretching, meditation, relaxation, purposeful breathing, and exercise is designed to enhance a mind-body balance. As an ayurvedic therapy, it is hypothesized to increase the body supplies of *prana,* which is a form of energy that flows (as yet undetected) through the universe and originates in the body during the act of breathing. From a less interesting perspective. yoga's mechanism of action could be subsumed under those attributed to exercise, stretching, and relaxation in general and would therefore be expected to confer some of the benefits attributed to these practices. Or, alternatively, its disciplined breathing activities could conceivaoly reduce stress by countering the irregular or rapid breathing associated therewith. However, as a CAM therapy, yoga is hypothesized to facilitate the process of unifying the body, mind, and spirit into a "oneness" that is capable of healing a number of diverse illnesses along the way. Where this "oneness" resides is not clear, but clicking Google's "I'm Feeling Lucky" option produces the Yoga Site, which in turn lists articles on how the therapy can balance the immune system, treat epilepsy, prevent hardening of the arteries, and reduce chronic pain. The Bikram Yoga College of India site (www.bikramyoga.com/Yoga/Benefits.htm) is a bit more specific with respect to the latter, offering the following guarantees for "curing chronic diseases such as arthritis or slipped disc":

> If you faithfully follow his directions, you will be relieved of your symptoms of discomfort. That is the only "cure" anyone can offer.

But Yoga offers two guarantees with the cure:

Guarantee One: If you continue to perform Bikram's Beginning Yoga Class™ regularly—all twenty-six poses—exactly as directed—the chronic symptoms will not return.

Guarantee Two: If you don't continue your Yoga faithfully, fully, or as directed, your symptoms will return.

Now that is an impressive pair of guarantees.

Herbalism

Also as previously mentioned, herbs are a major component of several medical systems. There are, however, CAM practitioners who label themselves "herbalists" and prescribe (and often sell) a bewildering array of botanical products and compounds that can be (and are) tailored to treat just about every imaginable human illness.

Given the number of these products on the market, no one can categorically say that none has any utility or efficacious chemical action. Nor can anyone say with certainty that some aren't actually dangerous for certain conditions or that they don't interact adversely with other drugs. More than likely a substantial number of the myriad herbs prescribed in a day's work by an herbalist have no positive or negative effects at all, other than the enrichment of the prescribing herbalist (and of course the corporations that package the herbs themselves).

Still, plants do contain chemicals, some of which are identical to those produced by the human body and some of which are identical to those contained in pharmaceuticals. Thus, there may be a "miracle" cure or two residing on an herbalist's shelf somewhere. How it could ever be differentiated from the welter of surrounding compounds that do nothing at all, however, is not at all clear.

Chiropractic Manipulation

On one level the proposed biological basis for this therapy is relatively conventional. It does not posit any unmeasured sources of energy, nor does it depend upon any new body systems. Few physiologists would also take issue with the importance of the nervous system—the chiropractor's locus of operation—in human health and disease. What is unconventional about the therapy's hypothesized mechanism of action is the large number of conditions that chiropractors consider to be due to the abnormal positioning of the spinal column, coupled with the argument that short manual thrusts can correct these abnormalities. It is these corrections, then, that are hypothesized to be capable of *curing* the diseases involved.

From a more transitory perspective, it is certainly not difficult to imagine that such a radical (and somewhat violent) manipulation of as large and sensitive a body system as one's spine could cause the patient to feel different immediately following the experience. This experience does not appear to *cure* anyone of anything, however, since it is reputed to be most rare for chiropractors ever to tell patients that they no longer need treatment for their ailments.

Spiritual/Energy Healing

To again quote Daniel Benor (who has written several excellent overviews of this field):

> Very sensitive people report being able to perceive these energy fields as auras of color surrounding the body. The colors shift constantly, reflecting the various physical, emotional, mental, relational, energy, and spiritual states of the organism. Particularly strong energy centers called chakras are visible along the midline of the body.... Healers find that the changes in the colors of chakras reflect states of health and illness in parts of the body near the relevant chakra, and that projecting healing to a chakra that appears abnormal can restore the energy to the body and improve health. The perception of auras is reported by healers even with their eyes closed.[5]

I include this long quote because I could never do it justice by paraphrase and because it might explain something about what happened once at my former CAM research center when a well-known healer was brought in to give a demonstration. A fellow statistician (and personal friend with whom I had worked for years) swore that she actually saw these auras emanating from the healer's body. I still work with this statistician, but only because she understands structural equation modeling and I do not. The fact remains, though, that *none* of the auras associated with these healers or their patients has been independently photographed. Nor have the energies emanating therefrom or any special gifts associated therewith been found to be measurable or observable using conventional scientific instrumentation—some of which, incidentally, is sensitive enough to detect the residue of energies that were emitted just a few seconds after the Big Bang. In all fairness, however, astronomers knew where to look for their energies, while conventional physiologists may have difficulty guessing from which body parts CAM auras are most likely to emanate.

Chelation Therapy

As mentioned previously, the hypothesized mechanism of action for chelation therapy involves an interesting twist. It applies a conventional chemical action based upon compounds, primarily ethylenediaminetetraacetic acid (EDTA), that constitute one of the few treatment options existing in conventional medicine for lead and other metallic poisoning.

EDTA is known to incorporate metal ions into its own atomic structure, but for it to qualify as a CAM therapy, the laws of chemistry had to be altered a bit. Hence CAM chelation therapists hypothesize that EDTA is also capable of removing a wide assortment of harmful ions, such as those associated with fatty acids—thereby serving as a potential treatment for heart disease, as a substitute for bypass surgery, or as a cure for a number of other ailments (depending upon what is being "chelated").

These proposed CAM benefits have yet to be verified, but this has not deterred an estimated half-million patients from receiving chelation via at least five million treatments. The average course of therapy is from twenty to thirty treatments, for an average cost of over $3,000.

Hydrotherapy

I haven't described this therapeutic genre before, but it involves the use of water, whether applied externally (spas, saunas, whirlpools) or internally (drinking, douches, irrigations), in the treatment of disease and injury. Many ancient cultures employed similar techniques, but the modern therapy itself was developed in eighteenth-century Germany—which perhaps should be called the fatherland of CAM (as well as CAM researchers). "Constitutional hydrotherapists" treat patients by wrapping them alternately in hot and cold wet towels and then applying a mild electrical current. Water, the most common chemical found in the body, is believed to relax (when warm), stimulate (when cold), and detoxify (through sweating or internal douches) the body. (In a sense homeopathy could also be considered a form of hydrotherapy since this discipline's medicines are nothing more than water with a long memory.)

Meditation/Mindfulness

One entire NIH-funded research center (located at Maharishi University) is largely devoted to the effects of transcendental meditation (TM), and I have personally sat through seemingly endless presentations touting the practice's curative properties. From a medical perspective, it isn't clear which biological mechanism permits meditation to cure disease, but its practice is hypothesized to produce a high state of central nervous system activity, which paradoxically permits a state of deep relaxation and rest. What this has to do with curing disease I'm not completely sure, which makes me wish that I had daydreamed a bit less during my Maharishi University colleagues' learned presentations. In general, whether it's TM (which belongs to a Vedic-inspired category of meditation that concentrates on a single thought or mantra) or mindfulness mediation (which has Buddhist origins and concentrates more on breathing and allowing the mind to simply observe rather than focus on whatever presents itself), I believe most therapists advocate the practice more as a lifestyle or stress reduction technique than as a medical therapy, which disqualifies it as a CAM technique.

Biofeedback

As previously mentioned, this therapy often employs the use of monitoring equipment to teach the individual to become attuned to his or her physiological functions (e.g., heart rate, electrical activity in the brain, skin temperature) and to ultimately control them in the absence of any equipment.[6] Biofeedback appears to be a form of relaxation therapy. Its basic assumption appears to be that many physiological components normally considered beyond conscious control can in fact be controlled. As discussed previously, Pavlov and his followers have definitively established that this can be done by psychological conditioning—hence there is no reason to question the fact that such control cannot be learned via other means. Like so many therapies, it is easy to see potential health applications of this technique, but unfortunately neither Pavlov nor any scientists who have followed him have seriously investigated any of these possibilities.

Hypnotherapy

Ever since our old friend Franz Anton Mesmer introduced the concept of hypnosis a few centuries ago, extravagant claims have been made regarding the etiology of the trancelike state engendered by therapists in individuals who are especially susceptible to suggestion. (Mesmer, incidentally, is mentioned with reverence among CAM scholars sans any reference to his ignominious experience with Franklin's studies discussed in Chapter 2. Now, however, the proponents of hypnotherapy have developed much more sophisticated psychological explanations for the phenomenon than Mesmer's animal magnetism, such as the "neodissociation model which proposes that the hypnotic process creates a temporary functional separation between certain cognitive control structures, resulting in the corollary separation of awareness."[7] I have absolutely no idea what that means, but it sounds far too impressive to be summarily dismissed. In any case, while hypnotherapy is often used as an adjunct to cognitive-behavioral psychotherapy, it possesses no generally accepted mainstream physiological mechanism relevant to human health.[8] Some work with PET scans has demonstrated differences between hypnotically induced states and general wakefulness in regional cerebral blood flow, among other things, but to show that hypnosis can make one less alert does not necessarily imply that it is a curative panacea.[9] Moreover, the introduction of a placebo has also been documented via imaging in a different region of the brain, which suggests that hypnosis and the placebo effect share a good deal in common. Both, for example, are so heavily reliant upon the effects of suggestion and belief that it would be hard to imagine how a credible placebo control could *ever* be devised for a hypnotism study, as witnessed by a typical preamble to a hypnotic treatment for pain:

> You've had such frustration, you must find it almost impossible to believe that anything can help your pain. It must be very hard to believe that I can help you. So it can be a very interesting, maybe very pleasant surprise when you begin to notice that you really are feeling better.[10]

Anyone who can distinguish between this quacking and that of the placebo duck is a lot more sensitive to animal sounds than your author. But then I never pretended to be a biologist.

Massage

In addition to the ancient forms of massage already mentioned, there are several far more popular schools or types of massage, most of which involve a therapist's use of hands either to knead tense body parts (Swedish) or to apply pressure at selected points that are hypothesized to be connected to important bodily functions (shiatsu). Personally I would categorize these procedures as more recreational than medicinal, since they are often used for relaxation and pleasure, sometimes employing fragrant and warmed oils. But some types of massage are more easily categorized as CAM, involving pressure (e.g., the Alexander technique) combined with specified movements or rhythmic rocking and shaking movements (the Trager method) that theoretically influence as-yet-unmeasured psychophysiological patterns in the client's mind. Most therapeutic forms of massage, however, are designed to attempt to help the body heal itself through loosening up muscular tightness and correcting other abnormalities found within soft tissues.[11] Hypothesized benefits range from stress and pain reduction to the improvement of immune function. Unfortunately, demonstrated health benefits are also hypothetical.

Magnetic Therapy

This therapy's origin has been attributed to Paracelsus (1493–1543), who reasoned that since magnets can attract iron, they should also be able to attract diseases and leach them from the body. While I certainly wouldn't question such a self-evident mechanism, I was even more impressed with Paracelsus' assessment of the role of the placebo effect in his new therapy, as reported by Vincent Buranelli in his history of hypnotism:

> The spirit is the master, the imagination is the instrument, the body is the plastic material. The moral atmosphere surrounding the patient can have a strong influence on the course of the disease. It is not the curse or the blessing that works, but the idea. The imagination produces the effect.[12]

This has to be the most eloquent argument yet recorded for the existence of a placebo effect, and it was formulated almost five centuries ago! Modern magnetic therapy proponents, on the other hand, have hypothesized a number of explanations for the healing results (which, as was shown in Chapter 11, are also only hypothetical). One physiological explanation involves the logical assumption that since iron is an important component of blood, magnets can improve circulation. Unfortunately, the iron contained in blood is of a form that is not attracted by magnets. However, other explanations abound—such as the possibility that magnets influence nerve signals, decrease deposits on blood vessel walls, and increase oxygen content of the blood. There's also the supposition that magnets must be helpful since the earth's magnetic field has been decreasing over the past century and a half. My daydreaming habit must have predated the above-mentioned Maharishi University presentations, since I can remember nothing from my physics courses that would explain the relevance of this latter fact.

Bodily Maps

This category of individual therapies has the distinction of having been heavily influenced by—some might even say having shamelessly borrowed from—the breakthroughs made by other CAM modalities. These therapies are usually based upon the notion that meridians or other conduits connect the different bodily systems (e.g., appendages, organs) emanating from a sort of circuit board located at a separate point in the body (although definitely neither the brain nor spinal cord). Given the fact that absolutely no physiological evidence exists for this conjecture, it is probably safe to assume that it will be some time before these hypotheses are validated.

Auricular acupuncture. The fact that neither the location of acupuncture meridians nor the energies that supposedly flow along them have yet to be detected by even our most sensitive instruments does possess one tactical advantage. Anyone can hypothesize their placement anywhere in the body that they please.

Paul Nogier, a French physician, must have learned this fact as early as the 1950s, since his seminal scientific contribution involved the realization that one of the unexpected functions of the external ear was that it contained not only a map of the entire body but also acupuncture points with direct connections to all of our bodily systems.[13] More precisely, Nogier noticed how the contours of the outer ear bear a resemblance to the shape of a fetus. Since there is no question that the fetus has (or is in the process of developing) all of the body systems and organs, Nogier—in one of the great scientific epiphanies of the mid-twentieth century—realized that the ear also must be connected to these body systems. Unlike many more mundane paradigmatic shifts (such as evolution or general relativity), this concept quickly caught on and was adopted by thousands of CAM therapists—even in China, the birthplace of traditional acupuncture.

To be technical, then, each body part has its own point on the ear, which in turn is directly connected to its own meridian; hence each point is capable of serving as a receptacle for a tiny acupuncture needle that in turn is capable of curing or ameliorating the symptoms of just about any disease or any part of the body not functioning properly. Auricular acupuncture, in fact, is hypothesized to work even more quickly (if that is possible) than conventional TCM acupuncture.

While not yet definitively confirmed by clinical trials (although, believe it or not, the *Archives of Internal Medicine* did publish one that didn't meet our quality criteria in 2000), the technique nonetheless has some very enthusiastic proponents.[14] I recall sitting through another interminable meeting with an air force colonel and the former director of the NIH Office of Alternative Medicine while the two of them tried to convince our center to submit a grant to the Department of Defense to develop auricular acupuncture procedures for the battlefield. The rationale was that while morphine and other opiates are undeniably effective in relieving pain, they have irritating military drawbacks (drowsiness and lethargy, among others) that pretty much preclude soldiers' continued combat participation while under their influence. Unfortunately, my center wasn't able to participate in this exciting project, which means that, for the immediate future at least, war movies will still resound with the call of "Medic, medic!" rather than "Acupuncturist, acupuncturist!" In any event, like other meridians, the existence of those emanating from the outer ear has not yet been documented, a small detail that proponents of auricular acupuncture tend to overlook. Perhaps when this therapy's biological mechanisms are found, they can either be evaluated (once biologists catch up with CAM practitioners) or, in the meantime, contrasted with those purporting to explain the placebo effect.

Iridology. First advocated by Ignatz von Peczely, a Hungarian physician in the nineteenth century, this school of thought holds that each body part is perfectly represented at a specific location in the iris of the eye. Hence abnormalities with, say, the liver should be reflected in the corresponding spot on the iris.[15] Peczely's personal epiphany came when he noted a pattern in the eyes of a man with a broken leg that reminded him of a similar pattern in the eyes of an owl whose leg he had accidentally broken as a child. I find this especially interesting, because while mouse, rat, and primate disease models are common in science, this may be the only recorded instance of an owl disease model resulting in a major medical discovery.

Not only has no physiological pathway been yet detected between the iris and other parts of the body, but the utility of the iris for diagnosing disease has been seriously question by controlled studies published in both JAMA and the *British Medical Journal*.[16] Experienced iridology practitioners were provided with detailed photographs of the irises of sick and healthy people in order to see if they could differentiate between the two. The therapists employed were unable to make such differentiations.[17]

Reflexology. This therapy uses the sole of the foot (and sometimes the palm of the hand) to model the remainder of the body. Tenderness or other sensations signal potential problems that some therapists believe can be ameliorated by massage—which makes this technique the masseur's analog to auricular acupuncture. And although the physiological basis for this therapy is about as scientifically well developed as that of auricular acupuncture, there are more than sixty reflexology organizations and associations listed on one Internet site alone.

Besides its use of a body map, reflexology also bears at least one similarity to iridology: controlled studies have shown that experienced reflexologists cannot reliably diagnose medical conditions by examining their patient's feet or hands.[18] Still, who says a practitioner has to be able to diagnosis something correctly to cure it, at least as long as the patient can be convinced of the cure's efficacy?

Intercessory Prayer

The final category of CAM therapies that I will discuss has the distinction of not merely stretching science beyond its recognized limits but doing the same with religion as well. Historically many indigenous medical systems—Native American medical practices being one of the more familiar—have used prayer (often quite ostentatiously) to effect healing.

Since there are few individuals still practicing these aboriginal religions in their original form, however, intercessory prayer as a CAM therapy typically employs individuals from a variety of religions to pray for unknown people's recovery, presuming that a single deity somewhere will respond. As the theoretical basis for these practices is theological rather than physiological, the plausibility of intercessory prayer is probably best examined from a mainstream religious perspective rather than a scientific one:

> In the major religious traditions, prayer that tests for response from God in the way the intercessor requires would not be considered prayer at all because it requires no faith, leaves God no options, and is presumptuous regarding God's wisdom and plan.[19]

While the evidence regarding these practices has already been discussed in the form of a negative Cochrane review (number 54 in Chapter 12), a more recent high-quality multicenter trial published in the *American Heart Journal* may be worth noting, since its results are relatively provocative.[20] This was a huge trial involving more than 1,800 cardiac bypass patients in six U.S. hospitals and partially funded by two Baptist organizations. The primary outcome was complication-free recovery from surgery. Participants were randomly assigned to three groups: group 1 patients received intercessory prayer after being told that they might or might not receive prayer (the usual experimental group), group 2 patients did not receive prayer after being told that they might or might not receive it (the usual placebo group), and group 3 patients received prayer after they had been informed that they would receive it (a very unusual group).

As is usual in the few multicenter trials conducted in CAM, there was no difference in complication rate between the experimental and placebo group (group 1 versus group 2). Surprisingly, however, the group that knew they were being prayed for did significantly worse than the other two groups. While this may well be a chance finding, there are several other possibilities. One is a negative placebo (nocebo) effect inflicted upon patients by the stress of knowing that strangers were praying for them. The other is divine pique at the presumptiveness of the researchers' belief that that God could "be compelled by our research designs, statistics, and hypotheses to answer our demand, 'Is the Lord among us or not?' "[21]

SUMMARY

So what's the bottom line? I think that most of us can at least agree that what we have here is a wide assortment of extremely creative therapies with even more diverse and creative hypothesized mechanisms of action. In some cases, these therapies ostensibly work by accessing energies, physiological pathways, and/or dimensions of existence that have not yet been observed, documented, or measured. In some cases we have therapies that borrow mechanisms of action from scientifically verifiable phenomena but stretch them far beyond anything recognizable by conventional science. In others we have therapeutic systems whose rationales were developed long before the birth of modern science but whose basic principles resonate with individuals who prefer ancient or exotic forces outside of our mundane existence—which perhaps explains why *yin* and *yang* or *vata, pitta,* and *kasha* are preferable to the earth, wind, fire, and air of ancient Greek philosophy.[22]

In a few cases we have therapies with elaborate and disparate mechanisms of action (e.g., yoga, tai chi, qi gong) that may provide health benefits similar to exercise and which probably are beneficial from a lifestyle perspective, as opposed to a disease-curative perspective. In others, such as hypnotherapy, hydrotherapy, and biofeedback, we have proxies for relaxation that, like exercise, probably have certain real, although quite limited, benefits. In still others, such as prayer, we have mechanisms of action that are borrowed from religious thought but are outside the purview of science. Finally, there are therapies that attempt to share their biochemical (e.g., TENS) or psychological (hypnosis) mechanisms of action with those of the placebo effect.

In no cases, however, do we have anything that would survive William of Occam's parsimony principle if we use the placebo effect as the comparator (or that would even survive the quacking duck principle). In truth, then, once applied to the proposed mechanisms for *any* of the therapies mentioned in this chapter, all that William's relentless razor would leave intact would be the one thing their use shares in common with the sole triggering mechanism for the placebo effect: *belief.* But the placebo effect has a plausible, empirically proven biochemical mechanism of action, while these myriad CAM therapies do not. Said another way, the mechanism of action of the former require few if any unproven assumptions; those of the latter requires a plethora of assumptions, some bordering upon the absurd. All of which leads to our fourth and final principle:

> *Principle 4: No CAM therapy has a scientifically plausible biochemical mechanism of action over and above those proposed for the placebo effect.*

Of course, just because there is no rational explanation for why something should benefit a medical condition or reduce a medical symptom doesn't mean that this something *can't* do so. Unfortunately, the results from high-quality randomized, placebo-controlled trials (Chapter 11) and systematic reviews (Chapter 12) have demonstrated that CAM therapies *don't* do so, which regretfully leads me to conclude that:

> *CAM therapies are nothing more than cleverly packaged placebos.*

And that is almost all there is to say about the science of CAM.

CHAPTER FOURTEEN

Tying Up a Few Loose Ends

While our primary mission has been accomplished, I believe we need to place our results into a larger context. Specifically, given the evidence that CAM therapies are no more effective than placebos:

1. Are there any other modern precedents for so many scientists in an entire area of endeavor to be wrong?
2. If so, do these incidents possess anything in common?
3. Could the public's access to scientific information be improved to prevent so many people from being misled by marginal scientific findings?
4. Ignoring everything said to this point, what courses of action are available to people who do simply want to find *something* that provides them symptomatic relief and who couldn't care less *why* it does so?

Earlier I artificially categorized inferential impediments into those affecting ordinary people, therapists, and scientists. While I did this in an attempt to make these rather abstract concepts a bit more concrete, ultimately we are all ordinary people and these factors conspire to help us all make fools of ourselves, scientists and nonscientists alike. So what I would like to do now is to examine a few relatively recent examples of science "gone wrong" to see if there are any commonalities with CAM research.[1] In doing so, I have leaned heavily upon three individuals who have put a great deal of thought into their explanations for how scientists manage to hoodwink both themselves and their colleagues: Irving Langmuir, Robert Park, and Christopher Toumey.

IRVING LANGMUIR: PATHOLOGICAL SCIENCE, OR THE SCIENCE OF THINGS THAT AREN'T SO

In 1953, Irving Langmuir, a Nobel laureate in chemistry, gave what must have been a very entertaining colloquium at the Knolls Research Laboratory. His talk was never published, but it was recorded and later transcribed.[2] In the talk, he discussed a number of blind alleys taken by scientists over the years because they failed to understand the importance of devising appropriate experimental controls. These oversights subsequently resulted in their perpetrators' seemingly complete inability to even consider alternative explanations for the accruing results.

In my opinion, CAM research is similar to investigations into the existence of extrasensory perception (ESP) and other paranormal phenomena: both types of inquiry, CAM and parapsychological, have enthusiastic advocates despite the absence of any physiological rationale for why such phenomena *should* exist. The concept of clairvoyance, for example, is eerily similar to some of the CAM diagnostic approaches whereby certain gifted individuals can sense auras emanating from diseased individuals and/or detect imbalances in their energy fields (or vital juices). To my knowledge, no one has conducted any scientific experiments to prove that these auras and their diagnostic apprehension exist, although during my tenure as a CAM research director I did offer to do so with the famous psychic diagnostician mentioned earlier who visited the center. For some reason she declined the offer.

Langmuir, on the other hand, encountered no such obstacles when he approached psychologist Joseph Banks Rhine (undoubtedly the most famous ESP researcher of all time) for an interview in 1934. Rhine, a professor at Duke University, was ecstatic at the prospect, believing that an encounter with such a respected scientist would greatly increase the visibility of his academic department.

At the time, Rhine was investigating both clairvoyance, in which he asked an experimental subject to guess the identity of facedown cards, and telepathy, in which he asked the subject to read the mind of someone behind a screen who knew the identity of each card. As designed, these experiments were quite easy to conduct and the results should have been quite straightforward, since chance occurrence was exactly 20 percent with the deck of cards that Rhine employed. Rhine's experimental procedures appeared impeccable as well, so short of fraud or some completely unanticipated artifact (such as occurred with the horse Clever Hans),[3] there should have been no way that the results could have been biased.

After conducting a huge number of experiments, Rhine found that his experimental participants correctly guessed the identity of the hidden cards 28 percent of the time. On the surface this may not sound earth-shattering, but then neither does the few centimeters of difference observed on visual analog scales favoring treatment over placebo groups in poor-quality CAM research. In Rhine's case, the sheer number of experiments conducted made the probability of such results occurring by chance astronomically low. In other words, it wouldn't be particularly rare for two or three experiments to obtain a success rate of 8% over chance (i.e., 28 percent minus 20 percent). But to obtain such an advantage based upon thousands of experiments by chance alone is, for all practical purposes, impossible.

After some discussion, and to Langmuir's astonishment, Rhine mentioned that he had filled a filing cabinet with the results of experiments that had produced only chance results or lower, and he took the precaution of sealing each file and placing a code number on the outside because he "didn't trust anybody to know that code. Nobody!" Rhine assured his interviewer that he was convinced these particular results were produced by people who were deliberately guessing incorrectly just to spite him. After a bit of probing on Langmuir's part, Rhine stated that the reason he hadn't included these negative results in his book on the topic was that he hadn't had time to digest their significance and, furthermore, didn't want to mislead the public.

Langmuir went on to provide a number of other examples of what he termed the "science of things that aren't so," including the reactions of their proponents when confronted by implausibility criticisms. One such example was a "well-thought-of French scientist" and member of the Academy of Sciences who thought he had discovered a new form of radiation (N-rays) based solely upon the belief that he had seen a brighter than normal spark using an elaborate but theoretically unsubstantiated piece of apparatus. When this finding couldn't be consistently replicated by other reputable laboratories (unless their scientists started out with a firm belief in the existence of the phenomenon), another renowned physicist traveled to France and discredited the entire field by secretly removing key elements of said apparatus without having any effect upon the occurrence of the phenomenon itself. In response, the French scientist said:

> That's one of the fascinating things about the N-rays. They don't follow the ordinary laws of science that you ordinarily think of. You have to consider these things all by themselves. They are very interesting, but you have to discover the laws that govern them.

All of which led Langmuir to conclude (and note that this is a transcription of a poorly recorded, informal lecture):

> The characteristics of [the examples he discussed], they have things in common. These are cases where there is no dishonesty involved but where people are tricked into false results by a lack of understanding about what human beings can do to themselves in the way of being led astray by subjective effects, wishful thinking or threshold interactions. These are examples of pathological science. These are things that attracted a great deal of attention. Usually hundreds of papers have been published upon them. Sometimes they have lasted for fifteen or twenty years and then they gradually die away.

Personally I think Langmuir was being charitable here, but this is as good an explanation of investigations and investigators gone awry as any. That the phenomena upon which they are based "gradually die away," however, is a fate that will probably never occur for CAM therapies because they have so many public relations experts working for them (e.g., the placebo effect, natural history, and cognitive dissonance), not to mention continued research funding from various sources, including the NIH.

Meanwhile, there is a happy ending to Joseph Banks Rhine's story, since the Rhine Research Center Institute for Parapsychology is still in existence and presumably still producing astonishing scientific breakthroughs. I even wonder if people don't remember the name of Joseph Banks Rhine more than they do that of Irving Langmuir. If they do, it is because Langmuir's seminal contributions to his field have helped it pass him by, while Rhine's field is in exactly the same state in which he left it.

In any event, based upon these discussions—all of which involved flawed experimental methods coupled with the fervent belief systems of their originators—Langmuir came up with what he termed a list of "symptoms of Pathological Science." Among these were:

1. The maximum effect is produced by a causative agent of barely detectable intensity, and the magnitude of the effect is substantially independent of the intensity of the cause. (What causative agent, for example, could be of lower intensity than a homeopathic remedy that has been diluted by a factor of several billion? And while the magnitude of effect is not independent of the intensity of the cause, it is negatively related, since the fewer molecules of the original substance, the stronger the effect. Or, taking intercessory prayer as an example, even its greatest advocates don't claim that longer prayers produce better results— although this philosophy wasn't shared by the Baptist preachers of my childhood as far as their sermon length was concerned.)

2. The effect is of a magnitude that remains close to the limit of detectability, or, alternatively, many measurements are necessary because of the very low statistical significance of the results.

(CAM effects are of notoriously low magnitude, even most of those emanating from low-quality trials. The presence of so much conflicting evidence in the research literature is another example of this principle.)

3. Fantastic theories are advanced to explain these occurrences. (This speaks for itself.)

4. Criticisms are met by ad hoc excuses thought up on the spur of the movement. In Langmuir's words, "They always had an answer—always." (One thing about the CAM proponents you may see on television or whose books you read: you won't often hear the types of irritating disclaimers that have cluttered this book, such as the three P's: *probably, perhaps,* and *possibly.* And you will never hear the phrase "I'm not sure.")

5. The ratio of supporters to critics rises to somewhere near 50 percent and then falls gradually to "oblivion" because "the critics can't reproduce the effects. Only the supporters could do that. In the end, nothing was salvaged. Why should there be? There wasn't anything there. There never was." (Well, CAM believers number well above 50 percent of the population, so the discipline may never fall to "oblivion" and its positive effects can be easily reproduced as long as a credible placebo control group isn't employed. I should admit, however, that I'm not sure about this prognosis.)

ROBERT PARK AND VOODOO SCIENCE

In an absolutely wonderful book that should be read by everyone interested in science, Robert Park discusses a number of case histories of individuals and types of research that traversed at least some distance along his subtitle's road (involving such disparate arenas as perpetual motion machines, cold fusion, and CAM) before arriving at a metaphoric crossroads:

While it never pays to underestimate the human capacity for self-deception, they must at some point begin to realize that things are not behaving as they had supposed.

Like all those who have gone down this road before them, they will have reached a fork. In one direction lies the admission that they may have been mistaken. The more publicly and forcefully they have pressed their claim, the more difficult it will be to take that road. In the other direction is denial. Experiments may be repeated over and over in an attempt to make it come out "right," or elaborate explanations will be concocted as to why contrary evidence cannot be trusted. Endless reasons may be found to postpone critical experiments that might settle the issue. The further scientists travel down that road, the less likely it becomes that they will ever turn back. Every appearance on nationwide television, every new investor, every bit of celebrity and wealth that comes their way makes turning back less likely. This is the road to fraud.

Few if any scientists are so clever or so lucky that they will not come to such a fork in their career. Almost all will acknowledge their error and put it behind them. Some will start down the road of denial but recognize in time that they are headed in the wrong direction and turn back. A surprising number—apparently unable to face turning back, and yet unwilling to follow the road all the way to fraud—seem to leave the road entirely, completely losing touch with reality. No matter how difficult it becomes to keep believing, it is easier than facing the truth.[4]

It is one thing for scientists to embark upon Park's nefarious road, but is it absolutely necessary for the public to join them? Since the public receives an abysmal scientific education in both the public schools and college, I think we have to look for the primary source of their information about science to answer this question. That source is to some extent the press, but in truth, its members receive no better scientific education than the public as a whole, so the scientific community itself bears some responsibility for educating the public. Consider Park's description of the OAM's 1992 press conference, with which I introduced this book and at which a scientific lunatic fringe was allowed to tout its favorite therapies to the American public under the auspices of the NIH.

Now, it may be unfair to fault the NIH for a press conference such as this, since it was forced, kicking and screaming, by political pressures to establish the OAM in the first place. Still, what more persuasive message could be sent to the public than that from an NIH-sponsored office confirming that there is a single entity called complementary and alternative medicine and that this entity should be taken seriously? The message was even more persuasive given that no one from NIH or the mainstream scientific community was at this press conference to offer an alternative viewpoint. Perhaps the presence of Senator Tom Harkin, introduced as the father of the legislation requiring the establishment of the OAM, would have discouraged that counterpoint anyway.

But the manipulation of the public's access to scientific information is hardly limited to CAM. Any scientific issue with financial implications (such as global warming or the health effects of tobacco) or religious ones (think of evolution or stem cell research) is subject to such machinations, often with the serious scientific community representing one side and pseudoscientists the other. In describing this phenomenon, I will draw on the work of someone who has a better command of the topic than I.

CHRISTOPHER TOUMEY: CONJURING SCIENCE

Christopher Toumey approaches science from a relatively unique anthropological perspective, and he has written a delightful book that explores numerous aspects of science's role in society, including how the public's understanding of scientific evidence is manipulated by proponents of various issues and how the press facilitates this manipulation.[5]

One of Toumey's most illuminating case studies involves the anti-fluoridation movement, which reached its peak during the late 1950s and early 1960s. While most people have probably long since forgotten this controversy, few public health issues have engendered more passionate emotions among so few as the introduction of fluoride into our water supply generated among the individuals who opposed it.

Without going into the historical details of these media-facilitated debates that Toumey so admirably describes, one method by which the antifluoridation movement attempted to sway public opinion was to people their press conferences with scientific "experts" whose expertise often had nothing to do with either fluoride or chemistry. As might be expected, these individuals were much more forceful than the real scientists who were called upon to present the other side of the issue. For present purposes, however, I think it is the lessons that Toumey draws from this controversy that are more relevant for us than the specifics of the issue itself. In a nutshell, Toumey suggests that the controversy was extended by the presence of two kinds of scientific corroboration.

The first was what Toumey characterizes as

> the pseudo-symmetry of scientific authority, [where] a small number of people with scientific credentials had more influence among anti-fluoridationists than did their colleagues who endorsed fluoridation. It mattered not whether the former were obscure, marginal, discredited, or numerically miniscule within scientific circles. It only mattered that they used their scientific credentials to extend the cultural issues into the scientific matter by saying in scientific language that fluoride was toxic.[6]

Similarly, the "science" of CAM was given a huge credibility boost by the very existence of an NIH CAM presence, even though the individuals initially funded by NIH (via its academic center grants) were better known as advocates of CAM than as first-rate scientists. In fact, one of the early directors of the OAM itself was an avowed homeopath. The awarding of these grants (always prefixed by the cherished acronym NIH) automatically bestowed scientific credibility on the advocates, as did their institutional affiliations, which originally included Harvard and Stanford universities.

To return to Toumey:

> The second kind of corroboration, the heavy weight of scientific uncertainty, made it even easier for science to affirm the moral values of the anti-fluoridationists. "Fluoride might be toxic"— these four words were more compelling than "Fluoride is not toxic as far as we know," provided that the former had at least a little grounding in some people's scientific credentials, some Greco-Latin scientific terminology, or some scientific citations.[7]

I have to confess that during my first meeting with the above-mentioned NIH CAM center grant directors I was extremely impressed with the erudition of these individuals and with their grasp of physiological terms, even though the terms didn't appear to have much relevance to the topics under discussion. With respect to the "heavy weight of scientific uncertainty," this refers to the importance of caution and evenhandedness that all legitimate scientists are taught, via the professional acculturation process (not to mention the peer review system), to bring to the conclusions they draw from conflicting evidence. Advocates, however, are convinced they *know* the truth and are completely impervious to conflicting evidence. They also tend to write much more compelling books than do scientists and are far more beloved of the media because, in Christopher Toumey's words, "good science makes bad television."[8]

While my personal experience with the media is not extensive, I have dealt with scientific writers from both sides of the aisle, both in discussing the results of my research (both over the phone to reporters and at news conferences) and also during my tenure as *Discover* magazine's methodological-statistical consultant. Based upon these admittedly limited experiences, it is my opinion that many reporters (scientific or otherwise) have not received a very good scientific education and have an absolute aversion to dealing with statistical concepts.

These deficiencies, then, coupled with externally imposed constraints that many science reporters find themselves working under, probably lead to the three characteristics of the press' coverage of science (articulated by Toumey based upon a book by Jerry Mander titled *Four Arguments for the Elimination of Television*) that encourage bypassing scientists in favor of quacks, advocates, and individuals with a financial interests when presenting evidence for or against an issue:

1. "Superficiality is easier [to present] than depth" (and people who have something to sell have an exceedingly simple agenda to get across).

2. "The media cannot deal with ambiguity, subtlety, and diversity" (which always characterizes scientific endeavors involving new areas of investigation or human behavior in general).

3. "The bizarre always gets more attention than the usual" (and things don't get much more bizarre than some CAM therapies).[9]

All of which leads me to a CAM example of the intersection of press coverage and advocacy: the glucosamine-chondroitin case study.

In her weekly "Personal Health" column published in the *New York Times,* Jane E. Brody does as responsible a job covering medical research as anyone, especially given the fact that she works on a weekly deadline. But in a March 2006 column, Brody takes umbrage with the large (more than 1,500 participants) glucosamine-chondroitin trial that, as discussed in Chapters 11 and 12, produced negative results.[10] Her primary reasons for disputing this finding (in order of presumed importance given her presentation):

1. It transformed her eleven-year-old spaniel "from an arthritic wreck into a companion with puppylike agility, giving him nearly six more active years." Anticipating the criticisms of naysayers such as your author, she further assured her readers that this

couldn't be a placebo effect since the dog had no idea what the capsules were and they were hidden in meatballs. Of course, she didn't mention the fact that the dog might have improved anyway, since we know very little about the natural history of arthritis in dogs, but that's a minor point. Or even that the dog might not have had arthritis, since the disease's diagnosis isn't 100 percent accurate in humans and undoubtedly is even less so in canines.

2. Based upon her single-subject animal study, she began personally taking three capsules of glucosamine and chondroitin daily (along with numerous vitamin and mineral supplements).

3. The capsules miraculously allowed her to continue to play tennis, ice-skate, walk three miles a day, and crochet—which leads me to question whether writing a weekly column is as time-consuming as I assumed. But this is certainly an impressive testimonial by someone the public has grown to trust over the years and who certainly can't be accused of having a professional or financial conflict of interest. There are the alternative explanations offered in some of the earlier chapters, plus the fact that all of that exercise might have helped her almost as much as her placebo capsules, but this is admittedly only speculation.

4. Appealing to authority, she mentions that her sports medicine physician reports that at least 33 percent of his patients have benefited from taking the capsules. (Which could be interpreted as yet another resurfacing of Henry Beecher's famous 35 percent estimate of the proportion of people who benefit from a placebo.)

5. Brody correctly notes that prior to the large *NEJM* study just mentioned, "two randomized, placebo-controlled trials showed that three years of glucosamine treatment slowed progression of arthritis on X-rays, as did a two-year trial of chondroitin sulfate." What she didn't report was any information on the quality of the three trials she entered into evidence, such as:

- All three were conducted in Europe.
- The first two glucosamine trials both lost over a third of their patients before they were completed.[11]
- The third chondroitin trial began with a whopping twelve participants per group, and its authors failed to mention if they lost any participants over the course of the study. This study's patients were also not blinded, and we don't know whether or not the individuals reading the X-rays knew which group the participants were in. (This is extremely important because otherwise it would be almost impossible for the authors to interpret the X-rays in an unbiased manner.)[12]

HOW CAN THE PUBLIC'S ACCESS TO RESPONSIBLE SCIENTIFIC INFORMATION BE IMPROVED?

We need to improve the public's scientific education, both in the public schools and in universities. Very few of even our best educational institutions (from the elementary to the postgraduate levels) give their students a solid grounding in the methods of science, but that is exactly what our schools should be teaching—that is, they should provide students with a firm understanding of scientific methodology so that they may then better judge the quality of scientific content, which is itself constantly in flux, that such methods generate. I would argue, in fact, that the epistemological principles presented in Chapters 3 through 7, not well understood now even by graduating Ph.D. students, should be introduced in the middle school years at the latest. If nothing else, understanding such principles might allow the public to recognize something like Jane Brody's recommendation of glucosamine for what it is—an attempt to manipulate public opinion through an appeal to authority with a little pseudoscientific window dressing.

I would further suggest that scientists have a responsibility to be available to reporters and scientific writers to help them evaluate the credibility and plausibility of scientific findings. (And print and electronic media executives must be willing to facilitate this process.) I would suggest that our funding agencies engage independent consultants—that is, scientists with no interests in a given trial's outcome—specifically to educate the public and help the media interpret the results of the studies these agencies sponsor. I would also suggest that governmental agencies such as the NIH do what they are supposed to do, which is to serve the public interest by advancing responsible scientific inquiry, uninfluenced by politicians and others with a decidedly unscientific agenda. And finally, I would recommend that scientists themselves get involved in teaching the public what good science is. I know every scientist in existence considers himself or herself to be extremely busy (and the vast majority really are, even your author), but we owe the public at least this much for allowing us the privilege of being this busy.

AFTER ALL OF THIS SOUND AND FURY, IS THERE NOTHING HERE TO HELP PEOPLE?

In truth, I don't know for *sure* that something like glucosamine and chondroitin can't be effective medications for something or someone. For all I know Jane Brody's dog will prove to be as important to the history of CAM as Peczely's owl. All I can personally do is evaluate the evidence that's available now and make the best inference its quality permits. As I've said repeatedly, it would border on the absurd for anyone to categorically state that among the thousands of substances advocated by CAM therapists and people such as Brody, a handful couldn't possibly possess some active (and beneficial) ingredients. Perhaps in time such evidence will materialize. After all, acetylsalicylic acid (aspirin), the first synthetic pharmaceutical drug produced, was based upon an active ingredient found in willow bark that was recommended by Hippocrates as well as reputedly used by several ancient cultures. And aspirin is now considered very close to being a wonder drug, although not necessarily in the concentrations found in tree bark. It has been said, in fact, that prior to the development of antibiotics, about the only effective medicines physicians had in their bags were aspirin, laxatives, and placebos.[13] But an isolated instance such as this hardly justifies the existence of an entire pseudoscientific culture such as CAM, any more than it validates the entire medical systems of the ancient cultures that employed willow bark for medicinal purposes.

But what about someone who is suffering from chronic pain and isn't satisfied with what modern physicians have in their bags? Someone who finds my final answer to the original question—whether CAM therapies are more effective than placebo—patently ridiculous and is now more determined than ever to try out a CAM therapy? There is an answer for such a person, and it resides in the research we reviewed in Chapters 9 and 10 involving the mother of all CAM therapies—the placebo.

HOW TO SELECT A PLACEBO THERAPY THAT WORKS

One thing I have saved you is the futile experience of going online to find out what does and does not work, which is the electronic equivalent of consulting a Ouija board. What you'll find there in the way of research evidence is a plethora of breathlessly positive studies conducted primarily by (or selected for presentation by) CAM proponents or studies that aren't positive but that have been given a little idiosyncratic spin by the Web site owners. These studies are small, of low quality, almost never placebo-controlled, and published (if at all) in marginal journals.

And what you'll find on clinically oriented CAM Web sites are the most astonishing claims imaginable, most of which won't be based upon any type of evidence (high- or low-quality) at all. Unfortunately, the few anti-CAM sites that you encounter may be just as biased in the other direction. Most problematic of all, you'll have no way to evaluate the validity of any of these claims, pro or con.

So how should you select a CAM therapy? First, before you reach the point of selecting one yourself, you really should consult your doctor. This suggestion may surprise you, especially coming from someone who avoids his internist like the plague and only makes an appointment under the threat of divorce court, but the fact remains that a qualified physician is the first person with whom you should discuss available treatments for your condition. Describe your dissatisfaction with the intensity or prevalence of your current symptoms and find out whether your doctor can do anything medically to relieve them. If not, that is certainly important information for you to know, and it is something that the two of you need to discuss *frankly*.

I italicize the adverb *frankly* because it would be a disservice to both you and your doctor to have anything but a frank discussion about your pain. Remember Dr. Smith's patients, who were too polite to tell him that his cherished therapy wasn't working? Politeness has its place, but not at the expense of your health.

Of course, the best-case scenario is that your physician will have a viable, non-CAM treatment option up his or her white sleeve. If not, what then? You should have an equally frank discussion about whatever CAM therapy the doctor recommends. Your valuing that recommendation will, if nothing else, enhance the you-know-what. But note: if you have a potentially life-threatening condition, don't discontinue your insulin, nitroglycerin, chemotherapy, or other treatment, because no CAM therapy is going to come close to matching these drugs' potency. Placebo effects are real, but they also have equally real limitations on how much can be expected from them. Neither a placebo nor a CAM therapy is going to cure anything that will not resolve itself or that the body does not have the capacity to deal with. Both a placebo and a CAM therapy that appeals to you, however, are equally capable of relieving pain if it isn't too severe.

If you're like many people, though, you won't ask for your doctor's recommendation and will hunt down other sources of information instead. Avoid the online route, as I've said. But you might scan Chapter 1 again and select the therapy that most appeals to you or, for a wider selection, consult one of the books referenced therein. After assessing what's available, you may want to select something that you can administer yourself, such as some herbs from the health food store or glucosamine and chondroitin from the pharmacy section of the supermarket. You *must* select something that appeals to you, however, because if you don't really believe the therapy will work, it definitely won't work. That is simply the nature of placebos.

If you prefer therapies that require someone else to administer them, then you're going to need to select a CAM therapist. You can ask your doctor to recommend a therapist, presuming that your doctor doesn't provide the therapy as an adjunct to his or her practice or doesn't dismiss it as an option. Or ask any of your friends who are presently receiving the type of therapy you've selected and get some recommendations that way. Chances are that a therapist who can elicit a placebo effect in someone with tastes similar to yours can do the same thing for you. Otherwise, consult the yellow pages and interview some candidates over the phone with the objective of finding one who is enthusiastic, who seems positive, and who has a personality that appeals to you. My only caveat here is that you should be mindful of therapists who can potentially do you some harm. If you are in need of, say, a chiropractor, you should check credentials and the name of the credentialing agency, and then look the agency up to make sure that it appears to be the therapy's primary professional organization. The help desk at your public library can facilitate this latter process as well.

Once you've started the therapy, embrace it and the therapist (the latter only figuratively) with all your heart and soul. Comply with the recommended regimen no matter how bizarre it seems. Also, be especially attuned to any advice that your therapist may give you regarding weight control, exercise, nutrition (especially reducing fat, sugar, and cholesterol intake), smoking cessation, reduction of excessive alcohol consumption, and so forth. Actions such as these may actually provide you with some long-term benefits.

After initiating the therapy, if you begin to experience some fall-off in its benefits, discuss the situation immediately with your therapist. Most experienced CAM therapists will have a menu of new strategies capable of initiating a new round of placebo effects. If none of them works, go back to the first step and repeat the entire process with another therapy.

MY WISH FOR YOU

If you suffer from an unrelieved chronic condition, I sincerely hope that you (or medical science, conventional or alternative) will someday discover something that will help you. And if the truth isn't out there yet and all you wind up discovering is some variant of Sarah's recurring placebo effect, I hope that the very effort of understanding your condition and the factors that tend to be associated with its exacerbation (and its ebbing) may be helpful and give you a degree of control over your life. I wish that, if nothing else, the hope that you will find something will itself be helpful. For the nourishment of hope is CAM's greatest strength. And the placebo effect is its sustenance.

Key to Abbreviations

Ann Intern Med   *Annals of Internal Medicine*

Arch Intern Med   *Archives of Internal Medicine*

BMJ   *British Medical Journal* (through 1988; *BMJ* thereafter)

Cochrane   *Cochrane Database of Systematic Reviews*

Eval Health Prof   *Evaluation and the Health Professions*

JAMA   *Journal of the American Medical Association*

J Clin Epidemiol   *Journal of Clinical Epidemiology*

NEJM   *New England Journal of Medicine*

Introduction

1. R. Park, *Voodoo Science: The Road from Foolishness to Fraud* (New York: Oxford University Press, 2000), 65.

Chapter One: The Rise of Complementary and Alternative Therapies

1. For studies by CAM-oriented researchers, see D. M. Eisenberg, R. B. Davis, and S. L. Ettner, "Trends in Alternative Medicine Use in the United States, 1990–1997: Results of a Follow-up National Survey," *JAMA* 280 (1998): 1569–75; D. M. Eisenberg, R. C. Kessler, and C. Foster, "Unconventional Medicine in the United States: Prevalence, Costs, and Patterns of Use," *NEJM* 328 (1993): 246–52; and J. Astin, "Why Patients Use Alternative Medicine," *JAMA* 279 (1998): 1548–53. Quote from Eisenberg, Davis, and Ettner, "Trends in Alternative Medicine Use."

2. For studies involving governmental and independent surveys, see B. Druss and R. Rosenheck, "Association Between Use of Unconventional Therapies and Conventional Medical Services," *JAMA* 282 (1999): 651–56; R. B. Bausell, W. Lee, and B. M. Berman, "Demographic and Health-Related Correlates of Visits to Complementary and Alternative Medical Providers," *Medical Care* 39 (2001): 190–96; H. Ni, C. Similie, and A. M. Hardy, "Utilization of Complementary and Alternative Medicine by United States Adults: Results from the 1999 National Health Survey," *Medicare Care* 40 (2002): 353–58; P. M. Barnes et al., "Complementary and Alternative Medicine Use Among Adults: United States, 2002," *Advance Data from Vital and Health Statistics*, Centers for Disease Control and Prevention, no. 343, May 27, 2004; L. Palamore, "Use of Alternative Therapies: Estimates from the 1994 Robert Wood Johnson Foundation National Access to Care Survey," *Journal of Pain Symptom Management* 13 (1997): 83–89.

3. Druss and Rosenheck, "Association Between Use"; Bausell, Lee, and Berman, "Demographic and Health-Related."

4. Ni, Similie, and Hardy, "Utilization of Complementary."

5. Barnes et al., "Complementary and Alternative."

6. L. Lao, "Traditional Chinese Medicine," in W. B. Jonas and J. S. Levin, eds., *Essentials of Complementary and Alternative Medicine* (New York: Lippincott Williams and Wilkins, 1999), 216–32.

7. J. Yang, *Zhen Jiu Da Cheng* [Great Compendium of Acupuncture and Moxibustion] (1601 A. D.; Beijing: People's Health Publishers, 1980).

8. D. V. Lad, "Ayurvedic Medicine," in W. B. Jonas and J. S. Levin, eds., *Essentials of Complementary and Alternative Medicine* (New York: Lippincott Williams and Wilkins, 1999), 200–15.

9. K. B. H. Cohen, "Native American Medicine," in W. B. Jonas and J. S. Levin, eds., *Essentials of Complementary and Alternative Medicine* (New York: Lippincott Williams and Wilkins, 1999), 233–52.

10. V. Badmaev, "Tibetan Medicine," in W. B. Jonas and J. S. Levin, eds., *Essentials of Complementary and Alternative Medicine* (New York: Lippincott Williams and Wilkins, 1999), 252–74.

11. G. Goodman, "Osteopathy," in W. B. Jonas and J. S. Levin, eds., *Essentials of Complementary and Alternative Medicine* (New York: Lippincott Williams and Wilkins, 1999), 289–303.

12. Ibid., 298.

13. M. T. Murray and J. E. Pizzorno, "Naturopathic Medicine," in W. B. Jonas and J. S. Levin, eds., *Essentials of Complementary and Alternative Medicine* (New York: Lippincott Williams and Wilkins, 1999), 304–21.

14. E. H. Chapman, "Homeopathy," in W. B. Jonas and J. S. Levin, eds., *Essentials of Complementary and Alternative Medicine* (New York: Lippincott Williams and Wilkins, 1999), 472–89.

15. D. J. Lawrence, "Chiropractic Medicine," in W. B. Jonas and J. S. Levin, eds., *Essentials of Complementary and Alternative Medicine* (New York: Lippincott Williams and Wilkins, 1999), 275–88.

16. D. J. Benor, "Spiritual Healing," in W. B. Jonas and J. S. Levin, eds., *Essentials of Complementary and Alternative Medicine* (New York: Lippincott Williams and Wilkins, 1999), 369–82, quote from 369.

17. E. Ernst et al., eds., *The Desktop Guide to Complementary and Alternative Medicine: An Evidence-Based Approach* (Edinburgh: Mosby, 2001).
18. Ibid., 2; E. Ernst, "Towards a Scientific Understanding of Placebo Effects," in D. Peters, ed., *Understanding the Placebo Effect in Complementary Medicine: Theory, Practice and Research* (Edinburgh: Churchill Livingstone, 2001), 246.
19. J. B. Moseley et al., "A Controlled Trial of Arthroscopic Surgery for Osteoarthritis of the Knee," *NEJM* 347 (2002): 82–89.

Chapter Two: A Brief History of Placebos

1. E. Ernst, "Towards a Scientific Understanding of Placebo Effects," in D. Peters, ed., *Understanding the Placebo Effect in Complementary Medicine: Theory, Practice and Research* (Edinburgh: Churchill Livingstone, 2001).
2. A. Harrington, *The Placebo Effect* (Cambridge, Mass.: Harvard University Press, 1997).
3. P. D. Wall, "The Placebo and the Placebo Response," in P. D. Wall and R. Melzack, eds., *Textbook of Pain* (Edinburgh: Churchill Livingstone, 1999), 1297–308.
4. H. K. Beecher, "The Powerful Placebo," *JAMA* 159 (1955): 1602–6.
5. S. Bok, "The Ethics of Giving Placebos," *Scientific American* 231 (1974): 17–23.
6. A. Hrobjartsson and M. Norup, "The Use of Placebo in Medical Practice—A National Questionnaire Survey of Danish Clinicians," *Eval Health Prof* 26 (2003): 153–65.
7. A. Hrobjartsson and P. C. Gotzsche, "Is the Placebo Powerless?—An Analysis of Clinical Trials Comparing Placebos with No Treatment," *NEJM* 344 (2001): 1594–602.
8. Ibid.
9. T. E. Einarson, M. Hemels, and P. Stolk, "Is the Placebo Powerless?" *NEJM* 345 (2001): 1277.
10. G. S. Kienle and H. Kiene, "The Powerful Placebo Effect: Fact or Fiction?" *J Clin Epidemiol* 50 (1997): 1311–18.
11. A. E. Shapiro and E. Shapiro, *The Powerful Placebo* (Baltimore: Johns Hopkins University Press, 1978), 41.
12. S. Stewart-Williams, "The Placebo Puzzle: Putting Together the Pieces," *Health Psychology* 23 (2004): 198–206.
13. P. Iacono et al., "Placebo Effect in Cardiovascular Clinical Pharmacology," *International Journal of Clinical Pharmacology Research* 12 (1992): 53–56.
14. E. P. Foster, *An Illustrated Encyclopedic Medicinal Dictionary* (New York: Appleton, 1894).
15. T. J. Kaptchuk, "Intentional Ignorance: A History of Blind Assessment and Placebo Controls in Medicine," *Bulletin of the History of Medicine* 72 (1999): 389–433.
16. Ibid., 396.
17. F. G. Miller et al., "Ethical Issues Concerning Research in Complementary and Alternative Medicine," *JAMA* 291 (2004): 599–604.

Chapter Three: Natural Impediments to Making Valid Inferences

1. M. Shermer, *Why People Believe Weird Things: Pseudoscience, Superstition, and Other Confusions of Our Time* (New York: Henry Holt, 2002), xxiv.
2. In a way this is ironic, but in this high-tech world, nothing is superior to patients' simple self-reports: not the observations of their physicians, nurses, or family members, nor the most sophisticated medical equipment.
3. R. Totman, *The Social Causes of Illness* (London: Souvenir Press, 1987).

Chapter Five: Impediments That Prevent Poorly Trained Scientists from Making Valid Inferences

1. All universities and accredited hospitals require their employees to submit their research plans to an institutional review board, whose purpose is to ensure that study participants' rights and safety are protected. Part of this process is an informed consent statement that each participant (or his or her legal guardian) must sign. This document explains exactly what will be done to the participant and what risks are involved therein. (As an aside, no one should ever participate in a research study who isn't given one of these relatively involved forms to sign. Furthermore, no one should ever sign one if he or she doesn't understand exactly what it says.)
2. Statistically and methodologically this is a reasonable practice, since including individuals who may not need the intervention (and hence cannot profit from it) is wasteful and mitigates against achieving positive results.
3. F. Galton, "Regression Toward Mediocrity in Hereditary Stature," *Journal of the Anthropological Institute of Great Britain and Ireland* 15 (1886): 246–63. (Or for a more readable account: D. L. Weeks, "The Regression Effect as a Neglected Source of Bias in Non-randomized Intervention Trials and Systematic Reviews of Observational Studies," *Eval Health Prof* 30 [2007]: 142–60.)
4. In recognition of these and other questionable practices, a group of clinical trialists, research methodologists, and biostatisticians came up with what is called the Consolidated Standards of Reporting Trials statement, whose primary purpose was to ensure transparency in the reporting of clinical trials and ultimately to improve the quality of these trials themselves. It now includes a twenty-two-item checklist that has been adopted by many medical journals and which can be used by their reviewers to "identify reports with inadequate description of trials and those with potentially biased results." While the adoption of these excellent recommendations cannot prevent dishonest or disingenuous investigators from lying about their methods, or putting a positive spin on their findings, their adoption by peer reviewed journals does at least ensure that the most relevant issues involved in the conduct of a trial are discussed. D. Moher, K. F. Schulz, and D. G. Altman, "The CONSORT Statement: Revised Recommendations for Improving the Quality of Reports of Parallel-Group Randomized Trials," *Lancet* 357 (2001): 1191–94.

5. K. Munger and S. J. Harris, "Effects of an Observer on Handwashing in a Public Restroom," *Perceptual and Motor Skills* 69 (1989): 733–34.
6. G. Homans, "Group Factors in Worker Productivity," in H. Proshansky and B. Seidenberg, eds., *Basic Studies in Social Psychology* (New York: Holt, Rinehart and Winston, 1965), 592–604.
7. R. B. Bausell, *Conducting Meaningful Experiments: 40 Steps to Becoming a Scientist* (Thousand Oaks, Calif. Sage, 1994).

Chapter Six: Why Randomized Placebo Control Groups Are Necessary in CAM Research

1. Random assignment entails allowing a computer (not the researcher or clinician) to decide to which group each person who volunteers for an experiment will be assigned. This helps to ensure that the treatment groups will be almost identical with respect to individual differences between people at the beginning of the study. People in my profession, in fact, firmly believe that one of the five commandments that Mel Brooks dropped on the way down the mountain in *History of the World: Part I* was "Thou shalt always randomly assign!"
2. This wouldn't happen in reality because, as will be discussed later in this chapter, his experimental participants would all be informed that they have a fifty-fifty chance of being assigned to receive fake (placebo) acupuncture. This induces doubt within the belief (or expectation) systems of both groups, thus dampening the placebo effect in both groups.
3. M. G. Fink et al., "Non-specific Effects of Traditional Chinese Acupuncture in Osteoarthritis of the Hip," *Complementary Therapies in Medicine* 9 (2000): 82–88, quote from 82.
4. Blinding clinicians is accomplished by not allowing the individuals administering the treatment to know the identity of the groups to which the participants have been assigned (which is next to impossible in treatments such as acupuncture or chiropractic). Blinding data collectors (or assessors) is accomplished by scheduling assessment in such a way that the research assistant collecting outcome data has no way to know which treatment any individual has received. Blinding statisticians is accomplished by having data entry personnel use a numeric or alphabetic code rather than the names of the actual treatment group (e.g., X versus Y rather than acupuncture versus placebo).
5. CAM is hardly the only area of medicine that suffers from these problems. In some surgical trials the placebo group involves nothing more than a superficial skin incision, which would take a firm believer in the tooth fairy to believe would fool most participants. (Which is not to say that credible surgical placebos have not been developed: some very creative ones have been employed.) To be fair, most CAM placebos are more credible than this, but this still doesn't mean that they fool a large percentage of people.
6. W. Rief, J. Avorn, and A. J. Barsky, "Medication-Attributed Adverse Effects in Placebo Groups: Implications for Assessment of Adverse Effects," *Arch Intern Med* 166 (2006): 155–60.

7. A. M. Brandt, "Racism and Research: The Case of the Tuskegee Syphilis Study," *Hastings Center Report* 8 (1978): 21–29.

8. R. J. Levine, *Ethics and Regulation of Clinical Research,* 2nd ed. (Baltimore: Urban and Schwarzenberg, 1986).

Chapter Seven: Judging the Credibility and Plausibility of Scientific Evidence

1. K. Dickersin et al., "Development of the Cochrane Collaboration's Central Register of Controlled Clinical Trials," *Eval Health Prof* 25 (2002): 38–64.

2. N. F. Col and S. G. Pauker, "The Discrepancy Between Observational Studies and Randomized Trials of Menopausal Hormone Therapy: Did Expectations Shape Experience?" *Ann Intern Med* 139 (2003): 923–29.

3. T. J. Kaptchuk et al., "Do Medical Devices Have Enhanced Placebo Effects?" *J Clin Epidemiol* 53 (2000): 786–92.

4. The effectiveness of these therapies was so obvious because the consequence almost inevitably and almost immediately followed the action and couldn't be attributed to something else, which makes for a much simpler inferential task.

5. CAM research is an exception because the National Center for Complementary and Alternative Medicine is charged with evaluating those therapies that are used frequently by the general public, irrespective of any evidence of plausibility.

6. E. Ernst et al., eds., *The Desktop Guide to Complementary and Alternative Medicine: An Evidence-Based Approach* (Edinburgh: Mosby, 2001).

7. R. B. Bausell, W. Lee, and B. M. Berman, "Demographic and Health-Related Correlates of Visits to Complementary and Alternative Medical Providers," *Medical Care* 39 (2001): 190–96.

Chapter Eight: Some Personal Research Involving Acupuncture

1. R. B. Bausell et al., "Is Acupuncture Analgesia an Expectancy Effect? Preliminary Evidence Based on Participants' Perceived Assignments in Two Placebo-Controlled Trials," *Eval Health Prof* 28 (2005): 9–26; S. Bergman, L. Lao, and R. B. Bausell, "Acupuncture as an Auxiliary Anesthetic for Dental Surgery," paper presented at the 2005 International Symposium in Oral Maxillofacial Surgery, Hawaii.

2. E. Ernst and M. H. Pittler, "The Effectiveness of Acupuncture in Treating Acute Dental Pain: A Systematic Review," *British Dental Journal* 184 (1999): 443– 47.

3. K. Linde et al., "Characteristics and Quality of Systematic Reviews of Acupuncture, Herbal Medicines, and Homeopathy," *Forschende Komplementarmedizin und Klassische Naturheilkunde* 10 (2003): 88–94.

4. P. Leggett Tait, L. Brooks, and C. Harstall, *Acupuncture: Evidence from Systematic Reviews and Meta-analyses* (Edmonton: Alberta Heritage Foundation for Medical Research, 2002).

5. L. A. Smith and A. D. Oldman, "Acupuncture and Dental Pain," *British Dental Journal* 186 (1999): 158–59.

6. The Jadad quality scale is a simple five-item checklist that allows one to judge the methodological quality of a trial very quickly by ascertaining if randomization was employed, whether the randomization was appropriate, whether double blinding was employed, whether the double blinding was appropriate, and whether some description of participant dropout was provided by the investigators. See A. R. Jadad et al., "Assessing the Quality of Reports of Randomized Clinical Trials: Is Blinding Necessary?" *Controlled Clinical Trials* 17 (1996): 1–12.

7. Ernst and Pittler, "The Effectiveness of Acupuncture," 447.

8. *De qi*, or needle pull, is a sensation experienced by the acupuncturist as the muscle "grabbing" the needle and by the patient as an electric current or aching.

9. S. Fisher and R. P. Greenberg, "How Sound Is the Double-Blind Design for Evaluating Psychotropic Drugs?" *Journal of Nervous and Mental Disease* 181 (1993): 345–50; C. M. Morin et al., "How 'Blind' Are Double-Blind Placebo-Controlled Trials of Benzodiazepine Hypnotics?" *Sleep* 18 (1995): 240– 45; M. Boasoglu et al., "Double-Blindness Procedures, Rater Blindness, and Ratings of Outcome: Observations from a Controlled Trial," *Archives of General Psychiatry* 54 (1997): 744–48.

Chapter Nine: How We Know That the Placebo Effect Exists

1. I. M. Klotz, *Diamond Dealers and Feather Merchants: Tales from the Sciences* (Boston: Birkhauser, 1986), 65.

2. S. Siegel, "Explanatory Mechanisms for Placebo Effects: Pavlovian Conditioning," in H. A. Guess et al., eds., *The Science of the Placebo: Toward an Interdisciplinary Research Agenda* (London: BMJ Books, 2002).

3. W. Lang and M. A. Rand, "A Placebo Response as a Conditional Reflex to Glyceryl Trinitrate," *Medical Journal of Australia* 1 (1969): 912–14.

4. A. Zwyghuizen-Doorenbos et al., "Effects of Caffeine on Alertness," *Psychopharmacology* 100 (1990): 36–39; M. L. Robinson et al., "Placebo Cigarettes in Smoking Research," *Experimental and Clinical Psychopharmacology* 8 (2000): 326–32; R. E. Meyer and Z. S. Dolinsky, "Ethanol Beverage Anticipation: Effects on Plasma Testosterone and Luteinizing Hormone Levels—A Pilot Study," *Journal of Studies on Alcohol* 51 (1990): 350–55; D. L. Longo et al., "Conditioned Immune Response to Interferon Gamma in Humans," *Clinical Immunology* 90, 2 (1999): 173–81; T. Luparello et al., "The Interaction of Psychologic Stimuli and Pharmacologic Agents on Airway Reactivity in Asthmatic Subjects," *Psychosomatic Medicine* 32 (1970): 509–13; S. B. Lyerly et al., "Drugs and Placebos: The Effects of Instruction on Performance and Mood Under Amphetamine Sulphate and Chloral Hydrate," *Journal of Abnormal Social Psychology* 68 (1964): 321–27; D. H. Bovbjerg et al., "Anticipatory Immune Suppression and Nausea in Women Receiving Cyclic Chemotherapy for Ovarian Cancer," *Journal of Consulting and Clinical Psychology* 58 (1990): 153–57.

5. Siegel, "Explanatory Mechanisms."

6. J. Matysiak and L. Green, "On the Directionality of Classically-Conditioned Glycemic Responses," *Physiology and Behavior* 32 (1984): 5–9.

7. N. Cohen, J. A. Moynihan, and R. Ader, "Pavlovian Conditioning of the Immune System," *International Archives of Allergy and Immunology* 105 (1994): 101–6.

8. B. E. Finneson, *Diagnosis and Management of Pain Syndromes* (Philadelphia: W. B. Saunders, 1969); C. Linde et al., "Placebo Effect of Pacemaker Implantation in Obstructive Hypertrophic Cardiomyopathy. PIC Study Group. Pacing in Cardiomyopathy," *American Journal of Cardiology* 83 (1999): 903–7; J. P. Thomsen et al., "Placebo Effect in Surgery for Menière's Disease. A Double-Blind, Placebo-Controlled Study on Endolymphatic Sac Shunt Surgery," *Archives of Otolaryngology* 107 (1981): 271–77; L. Cobb et al., "An Evaluation of Internal-Mammary Artery Ligation by a Double-Blind Tecnic," *NEJM* 260 (1959): 115–18; E. G. Diamond, C. F. Kittle, and J. E. Crockett, "Comparison of Internal Mammary Ligation and Sham Operation for Angina Pectoris," *American Journal of Cardiology* 5 (1960): 483–86.

9. C. G. Helman, "Placebos and Nocebos: The Cultural Construction of Belief," in D. Peters, ed., *Understanding the Placebo Effect in Complementary Medicine: Theory, Practice and Research* (Edinburgh: Churchill Livingstone, 2001); I. Kirsch and G. Sapirstein, "Listening to Prozac but Hearing Placebo: A Meta-analysis of Antidepressant Medication," *Prevention and Treatment* 1 (1999), article 0002a (http://journals.apa.org/treatment/folume1/pree0010002a.html).

10. A. J. M. de Craen et al., "Effect of Colour of Drugs: Systematic Review of Perceived Effect of Drugs and Their Effectiveness," *BMJ* 313 (1996): 1624–26.

11. T. J. Kaptchuk et al., "Sham Device v. Inert Pill: Randomised Controlled Trial of Two Placebo Treatments," *BMJ* 332 (2006): 391–97.

12. T. J. Kaptchuk et al., "Do Medical Devices Have Enhanced Placebo Effects?" *J Clin Epidemiol* 53 (2000): 786–92.

13. M. P. Jensen and P. Karoly, "Motivation and Expectancy Factors in Symptom Perception: A Laboratory Study of the Placebo Effect," *Psychosomatic Medicine* 53 (1991): 144–52.

14. G. E. Hogarty and S. C. Goldberg, "Drugs and Sociotherapy in the Aftercare of Schizophrenic Patients. One-Year Relapse Rates," *Archives of General Psychiatry* 28 (1973): 54–65; CDPRG, "Influence of Adherence to Treatment and Response of Cholesterol on Mortality in the Coronary Drug Project," *NEJM* 303 (1980): 1038–41; P. A. Pizzo et al., "Oral Antibiotic Prophylaxis in Patients with Cancer: A Double-Blind Randomized Placebo-Controlled Trial," *Journal of Pediatrics* 102 (1983): 125–33; R. Horwitz et al., "Treatment Adherence and Risk of Death After Myocardial Infarction," *Lancet* 336 (1990): 542–45; J. Irvine et al., "Poor Adherence to Placebo or Amiodarone Therapy Predicts Mortality: Results from the CAMIAT Study," *Psychosomatic Medicine* 61 (1999): 566–75.

15. Kirsch and Sapirstein, "Listening to Prozac"; R. de la Fuente-Fernandez et al., "Expectation and Dopamine Release: Mechanism of the Placebo Effect in Parkinson's Disease," *Science* 293 (2001): 1164–66.

16. I. Hashish, C. Feinman, and W. Harvey, "Reduction of Postoperative Pain and Swelling by Ultrasound: A Placebo Effect," *Pain* 83 (1988): 303–11; G. Remington, I. Fornazzari, and R. Sethna, "Placebo Response in Refractory Tardive Akathisia," *Canadian Journal of Psychiatry* 38 (1993): 245–50; E. Burunat et al., "Conditioning the Placebo Response in the Rotational Model of Parkinson's Disease," *Functional*

Neurology 2 (1987): 263–69; C. G. Goetz et al., "Objective Changes in Motor Function During Placebo Treatment in PD," *Neurology* 54 (2000): 710–14; J. M. S. Pearce, "The Placebo Enigma," *QJM: Monthly Journal of the Association of Physicians* 88 (1995): 215–20; R. Grenfell, A. H. Briggs, and W. C. Holland, "A Double-Blind Study of the Treatment of Hypertension," *JAMA* 176 (1961): 124–67; S. Carne, "The Action of Chorionic Gonadotrophin in the Obese," *Lancet* 2 (1961): 1282–84; T. P. Archer and C. V. Leier, "Placebo Treatment in Congestive Heart Failure," *Cardiology* 81 (1992): 125–33; D. E. Moerman, "Cultural Variations in the Placebo Effect: Ulcers, Anxiety, and Blood Pressure," *Medical Anthropology Quarterly* 14 (2000): 1–22; A. J. de Craen et al., "Placebo Effect in the Treatment of Duodenal Ulcer," *British Journal of Clinical Pharmacology* 48 (1999): 853–60; CDPRG, "Influence of Adherence"; Matysiak and Green, "On the Directionality"; P. Rosenzweig, S. Brohier, and A. Zipfel, "The Placebo Effect in Healthy Volunteers: Influence of Experimental Conditions on the Adverse Events Profile During Phase I Studies," *Clinical Pharmacology and Therapeutics* 54 (1993): 578–83; F. Benedetti et al., "Inducing Placebo Respiratory Depressant Responses in Humans via Opioid Receptors," *European Journal of Neuroscience* 11 (1999): 625–31; J. Oddmund, J. Brox, and M. A. Flaten, "Placebo and Nocebo Responses, Cortisol, and Circulating Beta-endorphin," *Psychosomatic Medicine* 65 (2003): 786–90.

17. K. B. Thomas, "General Practice Consultations: Is There Any Point in Being Positive?" *BMJ* 294 (1987): 1200–2.

18. This study was actually a little more complicated than I have implied, possessing two additional groups. I didn't think that these extra groups were really relevant to the present discussion, however, so I opted for simplicity.

19. A. Pollo et al., "Response Expectancies in Placebo Analgesia and Their Clinical Relevance," *Pain* 93 (2001): 77–84.

20. Does the 34 percent figure for group 3 sound familiar? It's not very far off from Henry Beecher's 35 percent estimate, is it?

21. Placebo research (such as the CAM research that I will review soon) is so voluminous that I can really only discuss what I consider to be the most relevant for the purposes at hand.

22. D. D. Price and H. L. Fields, "The Contribution of Desire and Expectation to Placebo Analgesia: Implications for New Research Strategies," in A. Harrington, ed., *The Placebo Effect: An Interdisciplinary Exploration* (Cambridge, Mass.: Harvard University Press, 1997), 117–37, quote from 127.

Chapter Ten: A Biochemical Explanation for the Placebo Effect

1. D. D. Price et al., "An Analysis of Factors That Contribute to the Magnitude of Placebo Analgesia in an Experimental Paradigm," *Pain* 83 (1999): 147–56.

2. D. D. Price, *Psychological and Neural Mechanisms of Pain* (New York: Raven Press, 1988); D. D. Price and M. C. Bushnell, eds., *Psychological Methods of Pain Control: Basic Science and Clinical Perspectives* (Seattle: International Association for the Study of Pain, 2004).

3. P. Iacono et al., "Placebo Effect in Cardiovascular Clinical Pharmacology," *International Journal of Clinical Pharmacology Research* 12 (1992): 53–56.

4. J. S. Feine et al., "Memories of Chronic Pain and Perceptions of Pain Relief," *Pain* 77 (1999): 137–41; B. J. Mathias et al., "Topical Capsaicin for Neck Pain: A Pilot Study," *American Journal of Physical Medicine and Rehabilitation* 74 (1995): 39–44.

5. J. D. Levine et al., "Role of Pain in Placebo Analgesia," *Proceedings of the National Academy of Sciences* 76 (1979): 3528–31; R. H. Gracely et al., "Placebo and Naloxone Can Alter Post-surgical Pain by Separate Mechanisms," *Science* 306 (1983): 264–65; P. Grevert, L. H. Albert, and A. Goldstein, "Partial Analgesia by Naloxone," *Pain* 16 (1983): 129–43.

6. T. L. Yaksh and T. A. Rudy, "Narcotic Analgesics: CNS Sites and Mechanisms of Action as Revealed by Intracerebral Injection Techniques," *Pain* 4 (1978): 299–359.

7. Levine et al., "Role of Pain"; Gracely et al., "Placebo and Naloxone"; Grevert, Albert, and Goldstein, "Partial Analgesia."

8. M. Amanzio et al., "Response Variability to Analgesics: A Role for Non-specific Activation of Endogenous Opioids," *Pain* 90 (2001): 205–15.

9. A. Pollo et al., "Response Expectancies in Placebo Analgesia and Their Clinical Relevance," *Pain* 93 (2001): 77–84.

10. Levine et al., "Role of Pain"; Gracely et al., "Placebo and Naloxone"; Grevert, Albert, and Goldstein, "Partial Analgesia."

11. P. Petrovic et al., *Science* 295 (2002): 1737–40.

12. T. D. Wager et al., "Placebo-Induced Changes in fMRI in the Anticipation and Experience of Pain," *Science* 303 (2004): 1162–67.

13. J. K. Zubieta et al., "Placebo Effects Mediated by Endogenous Opioid Activity on μ-Opioid Receptors," *Journal of Neuroscience* 25 (2005): 7754–62.

14. J. Kong et al., "Brain Activity Associated with Expectancy-Enhanced Placebo Analgesia as Measured by Functional Magnetic Resonance Imaging," *Journal of Neuroscience* 26 (2006): 381–88, quotes from 383, 386.

Chapter Eleven: What High-Quality Trials Reveal About CAM

1. The Cochrane Library, www.cochrane.org.

2. R. A. Davidson, "Source of Funding and Outcome of Clinical Trials," *Journal of General Internal Medicine* 1 (1986): 155–58; P. A. Rochon et al., "A Study of Manufacturer-Supported Trials of Nonsteroidal and Anti-inflammatory Drugs in the Treatment of Arthritis," *Arch Intern Med* 154 (1994): 157–63; M. K. Cho and L. A. Bero, "The Quality of Drug Studies Published in Symposium Proceedings," *Ann Intern Med* 124 (1996): 485–89; M. Friedberg et al., "Evaluation of Conflict of Interest in Economic Analyses of New Drugs Used in Oncology," *JAMA* 282 (1999): 1453–57.

3. W. Broad and N. Wade, *Betrayers of the Truth* (New York: Simon and Schuster, 1982); A. Kohn, *False Prophets* (New York: Basil Blackwell, 1988).

4. A. Vickers et al., "Do Certain Countries Produce Only Positive Results? A Systematic Review of Controlled Trials," *Controlled Clinical Trials* 19, 2 (1998): 159–66.

5. I wrote a book some years ago titled *Conducting Meaningful Experiments: 40 Steps to Becoming a Scientist* (Thousand Oaks, Calif.: Sage, 1994). The first step or principle was "Conduct your first research study under the tutelage of an experienced, principled mentor." The fourth principle, which I would now place as number one, was "Do not contemplate conducting research if you are not prepared to be absolutely, uncompromisingly, unfashionably honest."

6. K. F. Schulz et al., "Empirical Evidence of Bias. Dimensions of Methodological Quality Associated with Estimates of Treatment Effects in Controlled Trials," *JAMA* 273, 5 (1995): 408–12.

7. When research journals receive an article for potential publication, their editorial staff typically gives it a cursory screening to ensure that it is appropriate for the journal, then they send it out to three to five researchers in the author's field (often including a biostatistician) for review. These reviews provide a judgment regarding whether or not the paper should be published as well as extensive revisions and comments. This is sometimes called the peer review process in science, and, while imperfect, it is the best we've come up with yet.

8. D. R. Atkinson, M. J. Furlong, and B. E. Wampold, "Statistical Significance Reviewer Evaluations, and the Scientific Process: Is There a Statistically Significant Relationship?" *Journal of Counseling Psychology* 29 (1982): 189–94.

9. P. J. Easterbrook et al., "Publication Bias in Clinical Research," *Lancet* 337 (1991): 867–72; J. M. Stern and R. J. Simes, "Publication Bias: Evidence of Delayed Publication in a Cohort Study of Clinical Research Projects," *BMJ* 315 (1997): 640–45.

10. D. Rennie, "Thyroid Storm," *JAMA* 277 (1997): 1238–43; R. A. Phillips and J. Hoey, "Constraints of Interest: Lessons at the Hospital for Sick Children," *Canadian Medical Association Journal* 159 (1999): 955–57.

11. P. Tugwell et al., *Evidence-Based Rheumatology* (London: BMJ Books, 2004).

12. E. Garfield, "The History and Meaning of the Journal Impact Factor," *JAMA* 295 (2006): 90–93.

13. A. Michalsen et al., "Effectiveness of Leech Therapy in Osteoarthritis of the Knee: A Randomized Controlled Trial," *Ann Intern Med* 139 (2003): 724–30.

14. D. C. Cherkin et al., "Randomized Trial Comparing Traditional Chinese Medical Acupuncture, Therapeutic Massage, and Self-Care Education for Chronic Low Back Pain," *Arch Intern Med* 161 (2001): 1081–88.

15. M. H. Winemiller et al., "Effects of Magnetic vs. Sham-Magnetic Insoles on Plantar Heel Pain," *JAMA* 290 (2003): 1474–78.

16. Positive because if participants had discovered to which treatment they had been assigned by the use of another magnet or piece of iron, then the placebo effect would have been enhanced for those having a real magnet implant and destroyed for those who realized they had been assigned to the placebo group.

17. C. B. Begg et al., "Improving the Quality of Reporting of Randomized Controlled Trials: The CONSORT Statement," *JAMA* 276 (1996): 637–39. Later revised as D. Moher et al., "The CONSORT Statement: Revised Recommendations for Improving the Quality of Reports of Parallel-Group, Randomized Trials," *JAMA* 285 (2001): 1987–91.

18. P. O. Szapary et al., "Guggulipid for the Treatment of Hypercholesterolemia: A Randomized Controlled Trial," *JAMA* 290 (2003): 765–72, quote from 765.

19. A. Margolin et al., "Acupuncture for the Treatment of Cocaine Addiction: A Randomized Controlled Trial," *JAMA* 287 (2002): 55–63, quote from 55.

20. J. A. Tice et al., "Phytoestrogen Supplements for the Treatment of Hot Flashes: The Isoflavone Clover Extract (ICE) Study," *JAMA* 290 (2003): 207–15, quote from 207.

21. M. L. Knudtson et al., "Chelation Therapy for Ischemic Heart Disease: A Randomized Controlled Trial," *JAMA* 287 (2002): 48´–86, quote from 481.

22. R. C. Shelton et al., "Effectiveness of St. John's Wort in Major Depression: A Randomized Controlled Trial," *JAMA* 285 (2001): 1978–86, quote from 1978.

23. Hypericum Depression Trial Study Group, "Effect of *Hypericum perforatum* (St. John's Wort) in Major Depressive Disorder: A Randomized Controlled Trial," *JAMA* 287 (2002): 1807–14, quote from 1807.

24. P. R. Solomon et al., "Ginkgo for Memory Enhancement: A Randomized Controlled Trial," *JAMA* 288 (2002): 835–40, quote from 835.

25. Winemiller et al., "Effects of Magnetic," quote from 1474.

26. J. A. Taylor et al., "Efficacy and Safety of Echinacea in Treating Upper Respiratory Tract Infections in Children: A Randomized Controlled Trial," *JAMA* 290 (2003): 2824–30, quote from 2824.

27. K. Linde et al., "Acupuncture for Patients with Migraine: A Randomized Controlled Trial," *JAMA* 293 (2005): 2118–25, quote from 2118.

28. W. J. Rogan et al., "The Effect of Chelation Therapy with Succimer on Neuropsychological Development in Children Exposed to Lead," *NEJM* 344 (2001): 1421–26, quote from 1421.

29. R. B. Turner et al., "An Evaluation of *Echinacea angustifolia* in Experimental Rhinovirus Infections," *NEJM* 353 (2005): 341–48, quote from 341.

30. S. Bent et al., "Saw Palmetto for Benign Prostatic Hyperplasia," *NEJM* 354 (2006): 557–66, quote from 557.

31. D. O. Clegg et al., "Glucosamine, Chondroitin Sulfate, and the Two in Combination for Painful Knee Osteoarthritis," *NEJM* 354 (2006): 795–808, quote from 795.

32. J. M. Graat, E. G. Schouten, and E. J. Kok, "Effects of Daily Vitamin E and Multivitamin-Mineral Supplementation on Acute Respiratory Tract Infections in Elderly Persons: A Randomized Controlled Trial," *JAMA* 288 (2002): 715–21, quote from 715.

33. D. M. Eisenberg et al., "Complementary and Alternative Medicine—An Annals Series," *Ann Intern Med* 135 (2001): 208.

34. B. P. Barrett et al., "Treatment of the Common Cold with Unrefined Echinacea. A Randomized, Double-Blind, Placebo-Controlled Trial," *Ann Intern Med* 137 (2002): 118–24, quote from 118.

35. P. White et al., "Acupuncture Versus Placebo for the Treatment of Chronic Mechanical Neck Pain: A Randomized Controlled Trial," *Ann Intern Med* 141 (2004): 911–19, quote from 911.

36. H.-P. Scharf et al., "Acupuncture and Knee Osteoarthritis: A Three-Armed Randomized Trial," *Ann Intern Med* 145 (2006): 12–20, quote from 12.

37. K. Newton et al., "Treatment of Vasomotor Symptoms of Menopause with Black Cohosh, Multibotanical, Soy, Hormone Therapy, or Placebo: A Randomized Trial," *Ann Intern Med* 145 (2006): 869–79, quote from 869.

38. S. H. Yale and K. Liu, "*Echinacea purpurea* Therapy for the Treatment of the Common Cold: A Randomized, Double-Blind, Placebo-Controlled Trial," *Arch Intern Med* 164 (2004): 1237–41, quote from 1237.

39. B. Brinkhaus et al., "Acupuncture in Patients with Chronic Low Back Pain: A Randomized Controlled Trial," *Arch Intern Med* 166 (2006): 450–57, quote from 450.

40. J. Park et al., "Acupuncture for Subacute Stroke Rehabilitation: A Sham-Controlled, Subject- and Accessor-Blind, Randomized Trial," *Arch Intern Med* 165 (2005): 2026–31, quote from 2026.

41. D. J. Maron et al., "Cholesterol-Lowering Effect of a Theaflavin-Enriched Green Tea Extract: A Randomized Controlled Trial," *Arch Intern Med* 163 (2003): 1448–53, quote from 1448.

42. In addition to the twenty-two trials uncovered in the four journals that met our quality criteria, eighteen were found that did not (four with no placebo group, seven that were too small, three with a dropout rate over 25 percent, and four that failed multiple criteria). As would be expected, the results of these trials were much different, with a 72 percent positive result rate.

Chapter Twelve: What High-Quality Systematic Reviews Reveal About CAM

1. G. V. Glass, "Primary, Secondary, and Meta-analysis of Research," *Educational Researcher* 5 (1976): 3–8.

2. M. L. Smith, G. V. Glass, and T. I. Miller, *The Benefits of Psychotherapy* (Baltimore: Johns Hopkins University Press, 1980); G. V. Glass and M. L. Smith, "Meta-analysis of Research on Class Size and Achievement," *Educational Evaluation and Policy Analysis* 1 (1979): 2–16.

3. Actually, to be fair, Glass did advocate performing what he called sensitivity analyses, in which the results obtained from studies of high methodological quality were compared with those from low-quality studies. Medical researchers, however, are much more concerned with controlling the placebo effect (which does not even exist for learning and which is almost impossible to control in psychotherapy research).

4. M. Clarke, "The Cochrane Collaboration: Providing and Obtaining the Best Evidence About the Effects of Health Care," *Eval Health Prof* 25 (2002): 8–11.

5. I. Chalmers, M. Enkin, and M. J. N. C. Keirse, *Effective Care in Pregnancy and Childbirth* (Oxford: Oxford University Press, 1989).

6. D. Fergusson et al., "Turning a Blind Eye: The Success of Blinding Reported in a Random Sample of Randomized, Placebo Controlled Trials," *BMJ* 328 (2004): 432–36.

7. R. H. Gracely et al., "Clinicians' Expectations Influence Placebo Analgesia," *Lancet* 1, 8419 (1985): 43.

8. J. A. C. Sterne, D. Gavagham, and M. Egger, "Publication and Related Bias in Meta-analysis: Power of Statistical Tests and Prevalence in the Literature," *J Clin Epidemiol* 53 (2000): 1119–29.

9. R. B. Bausell and Y. F. Li, *Power Analysis for Experimental Research: A Practical Guide for the Biological, Medical and Social Sciences* (Cambridge: Cambridge University Press, 2002).

10. J. Ezzo et al., "Reviewing the Reviews: How Strong Is the Evidence? How Clear Are the Conclusions?" *International Journal of Technology Assessment in Health Care* 17 (2001): 457–66.

11. S. H. Zhang et al., "Acupuncture for Acute Stroke," *Cochrane* 2005, issue 2, art. no. CD003317.

12. R. W. McCarney et al., "Acupuncture for Chronic Asthma," *Cochrane* 2003, issue 3, art. no. CD000008.
13. L. He et al., "Acupuncture for Bell's Palsy," *Cochrane* 2004, issue 1, art. no. CD002914.
14. D. Melchart et al., "Acupuncture for Idiopathic Headache," *Cochrane* 2001, issue 1, art. no. CD001218; first quote from 7.
15. C. A. Smith and P. P. J. Hay, "Acupuncture for Depression," *Cochrane* 2004, issue 3, art. no. CD004046.
16. S. Green et al., "Acupuncture for Lateral Elbow Pain," *Cochrane* 2002, issue 1, art. no. CD003527.
17. D. K. L. Cheuk and V. Wong, "Acupuncture for Epilepsy," *Cochrane* 2006, issue 4, art. no. CD005062.
18. B. Lim et al., "Acupuncture for Treatment of Irritable Bowel Syndrome," *Cochrane* 2006, issue 4, art. no. CD005111.
19. A. D. Furlan et al., "Acupuncture and Dry-Needling for Low Back Pain," *Cochrane* 2005, issue 1, art. no. CD001351.
20. B. G. Haraldsson et al., "Massage for Mechanical Neck Disorders," *Cochrane* 2006, issue 4, art. no. CD004871.
21. A. R. White, H. Rampes, and J. L. Campbell, "Acupuncture and Related Interventions for Smoking Cessation," *Cochrane* 2006, issue 1, art. no. CD000009.
22. S. Green, R. Buchbinder, and S. Hetrick, "Acupuncture for Shoulder Pain," *Cochrane* 2005, issue 2, art. no. CD005319.
23. J. Rathbone and J. Xia, "Acupuncture for Schizophrenia," *Cochrane* 2005, issue 4, art. no. CD005475.
24. H. M. Wu et al., "Acupuncture for Stroke Rehabilitation," *Cochrane* 2006, issue 4, art. no. CD004131.
25. J. M. Ezzo et al., "Acupuncture-Point Stimulation for Chemotherapy-Induced Nausea or Vomiting," *Cochrane* 2006, issue 4, art. no. CD002285.
26. S. Gates, L. A. Smiths, and D. R. Foxcroft, "Auricular Acupuncture for Cocaine Dependence," *Cochrane* 2006, issue 4, art. no. CD005192.
27. D. Fellowes, K. Barnes, and S. Wilkinson, "Aromatherapy and Massage for Symptom Relief in Patients with Cancer," *Cochrane* 2004, issue 3, art. no. CD002287.
28. R. Ruddy and D. Milnes, "Art Therapy for Schizophrenia or Schizophrenia-like Illnesses," *Cochrane* 2005, issue 4, art. no. CD003728.
29. M. H. Pittler, J. Thompson Coon, and E. Ernst, "Artichoke Leaf Extract for Treating Hypercholesterolaemia," *Cochrane* 2002, issue 3, art. no. CD003335.
30. A. P. Verhagen et al., "Balneotherapy for Rheumatoid Arthritis," *Cochrane* 2004, issue 1, art. no. CD000518.
31. C. Norton, G. Hosker, and M. Brazzelli, "Biofeedback and/or Sphincter Exercises for the Treatment of Faecal Incontinence in Adults," *Cochrane* 2000, issue 2, art. no. CD002111.
32. T. Wilt et al., "Cernilton for Benign Prostatic Hyperplasia," *Cochrane* 1998, issue 3, art. no. CD001042.
33. M. V. Villarruz, A. Dans, and F. Tan, "Chelation Therapy for Atherosclerotic Cardiovascular Disease," *Cochrane* 2002, issue 4, art. no. CD002785.
34. H. J. Smith and M. Meremikwu, "Iron Chelating Agents for Treating Malaria," *Cochrane* 2003, issue 2, art. no. CD001474.
35. C. A. Smith et al., "Complementary and Alternative Therapies for Pain Management in Labour," *Cochrane* 2003, issue 2, art. no. CD003521.

36. C. M. A. Glazener, J. H. C. Evans, and D. K. L. Cheuk, "Complementary and Miscellaneous Interventions for Nocturnal Enuresis in Children," *Cochrane* 2005, issue 2, art. no. CD005230.

37. B. Wu, M. Liu, and S. Zhang, "Dan Shen Agents for Acute Ischaemic Stroke," *Cochrane* 2004, issue 4, art. no. CD004295.

38. K. Linde et al., "Echinacea for Preventing and Treating the Common Cold," *Cochrane* 2006, issue 1, art. no. CD000530.

39. C. I. M. Price and A. D. Pandyan, "Electrical Stimulation for Preventing and Treating Post-stroke Shoulder Pain," *Cochrane* 2000, issue 4, art. no. CD001698.

40. P. Kroeling et al., "Electrotherapy for Neck Disorders," *Cochrane* 2005, issue 2, art. no. CD004251.

41. J. M. Hulme et al., "Electromagnetic Fields for the Treatment of Osteoarthritis," *Cochrane* 2002, issue 1, art. no. CD003523; second quote from 6.

42. K. Flemming and N. Cullum, "Electromagnetic Therapy for Treating Pressure Sores," *Cochrane* 2001, issue 1, art. no. CD002930.

43. K. Flemming and N. Cullum, "Electromagnetic Therapy for Treating Venous Leg Ulcers," *Cochrane* 2001, issue 1, art. no. CD002933.

44. M. H. Pittler and E. Ernst, "Feverfew for Preventing Migraine," *Cochrane* 2004, issue 1, art. no. CD002286.

45. S. Meher and L. Duley, "Garlic for Preventing Pre-eclampsia and Its Complications," *Cochrane* 2006, issue 4, art. no. CD006065.

46. T. E. Towheed et al., "Glucosamine Therapy for Treating Osteoarthritis" [update], *Cochrane* 2005, issue 2, art. no. CD002946.

47. C. V. Little, T. Parsons, and S. Logan, "Herbal Therapy for Treating Osteoarthritis," *Cochrane* 2000, issue 4, art. no. CD002947.

48. C. V. Little and T. Parsons, "Herbal Therapy for Treating Rheumatoid Arthritis," *Cochrane* 2000, issue 4, art. no. CD002948.

49. J. J. Gagnier et al., "Herbal Medicine for Low Back Pain," *Cochrane* 2006, issue 4, art. no. CD004504.

50. T. Wilt et al., "*Pygeum africanum* for Benign Prostatic Hyperplasia," *Cochrane* 1998, issue 1, art. no. CD001044.

51. J. P. Liu, H. McIntosh, and H. Lin, "Chinese Medicinal Herbs for Chronic Hepatitis B," *Cochrane* 2000, issue 4, art. no. CD001940.

52. J. P. Liu et al., "Medicinal Herbs for Hepatitis C Virus Infection," *Cochrane* 2001, issue 4, art. no. CD003183.

53. J. P. Liu, M. Yang, and X. M. Du, "Herbal Medicines for Viral Myocarditis," *Cochrane* 2004, issue 3, art. no. CD003711.

54. J. P. Liu, E. Manheimer, and M. Yang, "Herbal Medicines for Treating HIV Infection and AIDS," *Cochrane* 2005, issue 3, art. no. CD003937.

55. J. Rathbone et al., "Chinese Herbal Medicine for Schizophrenia," *Cochrane* 2005, issue 4, art. no. CD003444.

56. J. P. Liu et al., "Chinese Herbal Medicines for Type 2 Diabetes Mellitus," *Cochrane* 2002, issue 3, art. no. CD003642.

57. X. Liu et al., "Chinese Herbs Combined with Western Medicine for Severe Acute Respiratory Syndrome (SARS)," *Cochrane* 2006, issue 1, art. no. CD004882.

58. W. Taixiang, A. J. Munro, and L. Guanjian, "Chinese Medical Herbs for Chemotherapy Side Effects in Colorectal Cancer Patients," *Cochrane* 2005, issue 1, art. no. CD004540.

59. J. Wei et al., "Chinese Medicinal Herbs for Acute Bronchitis," *Cochrane* 2005, issue 3, art. no. CD004560.

60. W. Qiong et al., "Chinese Medicinal Herbs for Acute Pancreatitis," *Cochrane* 2005, issue 1, art. no. CD003631.

61. X. Y. Chen et al., "Chinese Medicinal Herbs for Influenza," *Cochrane* 2005, issue 1, art. no. CD004559.

62. W. Zhang et al., "Chinese Herbal Medicine for Atopic Eczema," *Cochrane* 2004, issue 4, art. no. CD002291.

63. X. Zeng et al., "*Ginkgo biloba* for Acute Ischaemic Stroke," *Cochrane* 2005, issue 4, art. no. CD003691.

64. J. Birks and J. Grimley Evans, "*Ginkgo biloba* for Cognitive Impairment and Dementia," *Cochrane* 2002, issue 4, art. no. CD003120.

65. M. Hilton and E. Stuart, "*Ginkgo biloba* for Tinnitus," *Cochrane* 2004, issue 2, art. no. CD003852.

66. M. H. Pittler and E. Ernst, "Horse Chestnut Seed Extract for Chronic Venous Insufficiency," *Cochrane* 2006, issue 1, art. no. CD003230.

67. A. de Izquierdo Santiago and M. Khan, "Hypnosis for Schizophrenia," *Cochrane* 2004, issue 3, art. no. CD004160.

68. N. C. Abbot et al., "Hypnotherapy for Smoking Cessation," *Cochrane* 1998, issue 2, art. no. CD001008.

69. A. J. Vickers and C. Smith, "Homoeopathic Oscillococcinum for Preventing and Treating Influenza and Influenza-like Syndromes," *Cochrane* 2004, issue 1, art. no. CD001957.

70. C. A. Smith, "Homoeopathy for Induction of Labour," *Cochrane* 2003, issue 4, art. no. CD003399.

71. R. W. McCarney, K. Linde, and T. J. Lasserson, "Homeopathy for Chronic Asthma," *Cochrane* 2004, issue 1, art. no. CD000353.

72. L. Roberts, I. Ahmed, and S. Hall, "Intercessory Prayer for the Alleviation of Ill Health," *Cochrane* 2000, issue 2, art. no. CD000368.

73. M. H. Pittler and E. Ernst, "Kava Extract Versus Placebo for Treating Anxiety," *Cochrane* 2003, issue 1, art. no. CD003383.

74. S. Milazzo et al., "Laetrile Treatment for Cancer," *Cochrane* 2006, issue 4, art. no. CD005476.

75. L. Brosseau et al., "Low Level Laser Therapy (Classes I, II and III) for Treating Osteoarthritis," *Cochrane* 2004, issue 3, art. no. CD002046.

76. L. Brosseau et al., "Low Level Laser Therapy (Classes I, II and III) for Treating Rheumatoid Arthritis," *Cochrane* 2005, issue 4, art. no. CD002049.

77. A. D. Furlan et al., "Massage for Low-Back Pain," *Cochrane* 2002, issue 2, art. no. CD001929.

78. N. Viggo Hansen, T. Jorgensen, and L. Ortenblad, "Massage and Touch for Dementia," *Cochrane* 2006, issue 4.

79. K. V. Trinh et al., "Acupuncture for Neck Disorders," *Cochrane* 2006, issue 4, art. no. CD004870.

80. T. Krisanaprakornkit et al., "Meditation Therapy for Anxiety Disorders," *Cochrane* 2006, issue 1, art. no. CD004998.

81. A. Rambaldi and C. Gluud, "S-adenosyl-L-methionine for Alcoholic Liver Diseases," *Cochrane* 2001, issue 4, art. no. CD002235.

82. S. Beamon et al., "Speleotherapy for Asthma," *Cochrane* 2001, issue 2, art. no. CD001741.

83. W. J. J. Assendelft et al., "Spinal Manipulative Therapy for Low-Back Pain," *Cochrane* 2004, issue 1, art. no. CD000447.

84. M. L. Proctor et al., "Spinal Manipulation for Primary and Secondary Dysmenorrhoea," *Cochrane* 2001, issue 4, art. no. CD002119.

85. G. Bronfort et al., "Non-invasive Physical Treatments for Chronic/Recurrent Headache," *Cochrane* 2004, issue 3, art. no. CD001878.

86. M. A. Hondras, K. Linde, and A. P. Jones, "Manual Therapy for Asthma," *Cochrane* 2005, issue 2, art. no. CD001002.

87. A. Rambaldi et al., "Milk Thistle for Alcoholic and/or Hepatitis B or C Virus Liver Diseases," *Cochrane* 2005, issue 2, art. no. CD003620.

88. A. C. Vink et al., "Music Therapy for People with Dementia," *Cochrane* 2003, issue 4, art. no. CD003477.

89. C. Gold et al., "Music Therapy for Schizophrenia or Schizophrenia-like Illnesses," *Cochrane* 2005, issue 2, art. no. CD004025.

90. S. Dagenais et al., "Prolotherapy Injections for Chronic Low-Back Pain," *Cochrane* 2006, issue 4, art. no. CD004059.

91. K. Linde et al., "St. John's Wort for Depression," *Cochrane* 2005, issue 3, art. no. CD000448.

92. T. Wilt, A. Ishani, and R. MacDonald, "*Serenoa repens* for Benign Prostatic Hyperplasia," *Cochrane* 2002, issue 3, art. no. CD001423.

93. A. Han et al., "Tai Chi for Treating Rheumatoid Arthritis," *Cochrane* 2004, issue 3, art. no. CD004849.

94. D. A. W. M. Van der Windt et al., "Therapeutic Ultrasound for Acute Ankle Sprains," *Cochrane* 2002, issue 1, art. no. CD001250.

95. A. Baba-Akbari Sari et al., "Therapeutic Ultrasound for Pressure Ulcers," *Cochrane* 2000, issue 4, art. no. CD001275.

96. V. A. Robinson et al., "Therapeutic Ultrasound for Osteoarthritis of the Knee," *Cochrane* 2001, issue 3, art. no. CD003132.

97. E. J. C. Hay-Smith, "Therapeutic Ultrasound for Postpartum Perineal Pain and Dyspareunia," *Cochrane* 1998, issue 3, art. no. CD000495.

98. L. Casimiro et al., "Therapeutic Ultrasound for the Treatment of Rheumatoid Arthritis," *Cochrane* 2002, issue 3, art. no. CD003787.

99. K. Flemming and N. Cullum, "Therapeutic Ultrasound for Venous Leg Ulcers," *Cochrane* 2000, issue 4, art. no. CD001180.

100. J. L. R. Martin et al., "Transcranial Magnetic Stimulation for the Treatment of Obsessive-Compulsive Disorder," *Cochrane* 2003, issue 2, art. no. CD003387.

101. J. L. R. Martin et al., "Transcranial Magnetic Stimulation for Treating Depression," *Cochrane* 2001, issue 4, art. no. CD003493.

102. M. Osiri et al., "Transcutaneous Electrical Nerve Stimulation for Knee Osteoarthritis," *Cochrane* 2000, issue 4, art. no. CD002823.

103. A. Khadilkar et al., "Transcutaneous Electrical Nerve Stimulation (TENS) for Chronic Low-Back Pain," *Cochrane* 2005, issue 3, art. no. CD003008.

104. D. Carroll et al., "Transcutaneous Electrical Nerve Stimulation (TENS) for Chronic Pain," *Cochrane* 2000, issue 4, art. no. CD003222.

105. M. Cameron, E. Lonergan, and H. Lee, "Transcutaneous Electrical Nerve Stimulation (TENS) for Dementia," *Cochrane* 2003, issue 3, art. no. CD004032.

106. L. Brosseau et al., "Transcutaneous Electrical Nerve Stimulation (TENS) for the Treatment of Rheumatoid Arthritis in the Hand," *Cochrane* 2003, issue 2, art. no. CD004377.

107. M. L. Proctor et al., "Transcutaneous Electrical Nerve Stimulation and Acupuncture for Primary Dysmenorrhoea," *Cochrane* 2002, issue 1, art. no. CD002123.

108. Basically there were four trials: two found in favor of TT, and two in favor of the control group (one significantly so).

109. D. P. O'Mathuna and R. L. Ashford, "Therapeutic Touch for Healing Acute Wounds," *Cochrane* 2003, issue 4, art. no. CD002766.

110. M. W. Lipsey and D. B. Wilson, "Educational and Behavioral Treatment: Confirmation from Meta-analysis," *American Psychologist* 48 (1993): 1181–209.

111. K. Linde et al., "Are the Clinical Effects of Homeopathy Placebo Effects? A Meta-analysis of Placebo-Controlled Trials," *Lancet* 350 (1997): 834–43, quote from 834.

112. Ibid., 841.

113. E. Ernst, "A Systematic Review of Systematic Reviews of Homeopathy," *British Journal of Clinical Pharmacology* 54 (2002): 577–82, quote from 577.

114. J. Barnes, K. L. Resch, and E. Ernst, "Homeopathy for Postoperative Ileus," *Journal of Clinical Gastroenterology* 25 (1997): 628–33.

115. E. Ernst, "Re-analysis of Previous Meta-analysis of Clinical Trials of Homeopathy," *J Clin Epidemiol* 53 (2000): 1188; K. Linde et al., "Impact of Study Quality on Outcome in Placebo Controlled Trials of Homeopathy," *J Clin Epidemiol* 52 (1999): 631–36; K. Linde and D. Melchart, "Randomized Controlled Trials of Individualised Homeopathy: A State-of-the-Art Review," *Journal of Alternative and Complementary Medicine* 4 (1999): 371–388.

116. E. Ernst and M. H. Pitter, "Re-analysis of Previous Meta-analysis of Clinical Trials of Homeopathy," *Journal of Experimental Epidemiology* 53, 11 (2000): 1188.

117. T. E. Towheed et al., "Glucosamine Therapy for Treating Osteoarthritis," *Cochrane* 2001, issue 1, art. no. CD002946.

118. T. E. Towheed et al., "Glucosamine Therapy for Treating Osteoarthritis" [update], *Cochrane* 2005, issue 2, art. no. CD002946

119. T. McAlindon et al., "Effectiveness of Glucosamine for Symptoms of Knee Osteoarthritis: Results from an Internet-Based Randomized Double-Blind Controlled Trial," *American Journal of Medicine* 117 (2004): 643–49; I. Ciebere et al., "Randomized, Double-Blind, Placebo-Controlled Glucosamine Discontinuation Trial in Knee Arthritis," *Arthritis and Rheumatism* 51 (2004): 738–45.

120. P. Hughes and A. Carr, "A Randomized, Double-Blind, Placebo-Controlled Trial of Glucosamine Sulphate as an Analgesic in Osteoarthritis of the Knee," *Rheumatology* 41 (2002): 279–84; J. P. Rindone et al., "Randomized, Controlled Trial of Glucosamine for Treating Osteoarthritis of the Knee," *Western Journal of Medicine* 172 (2000): 91–94.

121. McAlindon et al., "Effectiveness of Glucosamine," quote from 643.

122. Ciebere et al., "Randomized, Double-Blind, Placebo-Controlled Glucosamine Discontinuation," quote from 738.

123. Hughes and Carr, "A Randomized, Double-Blind, Placebo-Controlled Trial of Glucosamine Sulphate," quote from 279.

124. Rindone et al., "Randomized, Controlled Trial of Glucosamine," quote from 91.

125. D. O. Clegg et al., "Glucosamine, Chondroitin Sulfate, and the Two in Combination for Painful Knee Osteoarthritis," *NEJM* 354 (2006): 795–808, quote from 795.

126. S. Reichenbach et al., "Meta-analysis: Chondroitin for Osteoarthritis of the Knee or Hip," *Annals of Internal Medicine* 146, 8 (2007): 580–90, quote from 580.

Chapter Thirteen: How CAM Therapies Are Hypothesized to Work

1. I include the disclaimer "established" because to survive economically a CAM therapy must possess enough *credibility* to persuade a reasonable number of individuals to continue to pay therapists or to purchase the ingredients necessary for self-administration—an application of the "survival of the fittest" concept that I seriously doubt Charles Darwin anticipated.

2. G. G. Zhang et al., "The Variability of TCM Pattern Diagnosis and Herbal Prescription on Rheumatoid Arthritis Patients," *Alternative Therapies in Health and Medicine* 10 (2004): 58–63.

3. E. J. Mayer, D. D. Price, and A. Rafii, "Antagonism of Acupuncture Analgesia in Man by the Narcotic Antagonist Naloxone," *Brain Research* 121 (1977): 368–72; J. S. Han, "Acupuncture: Neuropeptide Release Produced by Electrical Stimulation of Different Frequencies," *Trends in Neurosciences* 26 (2003): 17–22.

4. G. Goodman, "Osteopathy," in W. B. Jonas and J. S. Levin, eds., *Essentials of Complementary and Alternative Medicine* (New York: Lippincott Williams and Wilkins, 1999), 289–303.

5. D. J. Benor, "Spiritual Healing," in W. B. Jonas and J. S. Levin, eds., *Essentials of Complementary and Alternative Medicine* (New York: Lippincott Williams and Wilkins, 1999), 369–82, quote from 377.

6. J. A. Green and R. Shellenberger, "Biofeedback Therapy," in W. B. Jonas and J. S. Levin, eds., *Essentials of Complementary and Alternative Medicine* (New York: Lippincott Williams and Wilkins, 1999), 410–25.

7. J. Barber, "Hypnotic Analgesia: Mechanisms of Action and Clinical Applications," in D. D. Price and M. C. Bushnell, eds., *Psychological Methods of Pain Control: Basic Science and Clinical Perspectives* (Seattle: International Association for the Study of Pain, 2004), 269–300.

8. I. Kirsch, G. Montgomery, and G. Sapirstein, "Hypnosis as an Adjunct to Cognitive-Behavioral Psychotherapy," *International Journal of Clinical and Experimental Hypnosis* 48 (2000): 154–69.

9. P. Rainville et al., "Hypnosis Modulates Activity in Brain Structures Involved in the Regulation of Consciousness," *Journal of Cognitive Neuroscience* 14 (2002): 1–15.

10. Barber, "Hypnotic Analgesia," 292.

11. T. Field, "Massage Therapy," in W. B. Jonas and J. S. Levin, eds., *Essentials of Complementary and Alternative Medicine* (New York: Lippincott Williams and Wilkins, 1999), 383–91.

12. V. Buranelli, *The Wizard from Vienna* (New York: Coward, McCann & Geoghegan, 1975), 20.

13. H. Huang, trans., *Ear Acupuncture: A Chinese Medical Report* (Emmaus, Penn.: Rodale Press, 1974).
14. S. K. Avants et al., "A Randomized Controlled Trial of Auricular Acupuncture for Cocaine Dependence," *Arch Intern Med* 160 (2000): 2305–12.
15. P. Knipschild, "Looking for Gall Bladder Disease in the Patient's Iris," *BMJ* 297 (1988): 1578–81.
16. A. Simon, D. M. Worthen, and J. A. Mitas, "An Evaluation of Iridology," *JAMA* 242 (1979): 1385–87; Knipschild, "Looking."
17. Zhang et al., "The Variability of TCM."
18. A. R. White et al., "A Blinded Investigation into the Accuracy of Reflexology Charts," *Complementary Therapies in Medicine* 8 (2000): 166–72.
19. J. R. Chibnall, J. M. Jeral, and J. J. Cerullo, "Experiments on Distant Intercessory Prayer: God, Science, and the Lesson of Massah," *Arch Intern Med* 161 (2001): 2529–36, quote from 2531.
20. H. Benson et al., "Study of the Therapeutic Effects of Intercessory Prayer (STEP) in Cardiac Bypass Patients: A Multicenter Randomized Trial of Uncertainty and Certainty of Receiving Intercessory Prayer," *American Heart Journal* 151 (2006): 934–42.
21. Chibnall, Jeral, and Cerullo, "Experiments," quote from 2535; Benson et al., "Study."
22. T. Marks, "Elemental: The Four Elements," http://www.geocities.com/tmartiac// myth/elemental.htm. It is interesting, however, that three of the five primary elements in TCM are earth, fire, and air as well, and these plus wind did influence both Hippocrates (the father of modern conventional medicine) and Jung (one of the founders of modern psychiatry), but that is grist for other stories.

Chapter Fourteen: Tying Up a Few Loose Ends

1. For anyone who wants to go back to the last half of the nineteenth century for an example, Stephen Jay Gould in *The Mismeasure of Man* (New York: Norton, 1981) provides an excellent history of craniometry, which was used to explain why women and blacks were inferior intellectually to white males of western European descent. Untold numbers of scientific papers and numerous books were written on the topic before the entire discipline disappeared in the twentieth century.
2. "Langmuir's Talk on Pathological Science (December 18, 1953)," Web site of Kenneth Steiglitz, http://www.cs.princeton.edu/~ken/Langmuir/langmuir.htm.
3. This horse became a major celebrity in Berlin around the turn of the century. The horse could apparently solve math problems; he provided the answer by beginning to paw the ground with his hoof, usually stopping at the correct answer, which no one could explain until an early research methodologist (at least that's the job title I'd give him) demonstrated that Hans couldn't solve the problem if his questioner wasn't capable of providing any sort of physiological or postural cue to tip Hans off as to when to stop his pawing behavior.
4. R. Park, *Voodoo Science: The Road from Foolishness to Fraud* (New York: Oxford University Press, 2000), 211–12.
5. C. P. Toumey, *Conjuring Science* (New Brunswick, N. J.: Rutgers University Press, 1996).
6. Ibid., 80.

7. Ibid.

8. Ibid., 56.

9. Ibid., quoting J. Mander, *Four Arguments for the Elimination of Television* (New York: Quill, 1978), 223–28.

10. J. E. Brody, "Fine Print Sends Clear Message: Stay the Course," *New York Times,* March 14, 2006.

11. J. Y. Reginster et al., "Long-Term Effects of Glucosamine Sulphate on Osteoarthritis Progression: A Randomized, Placebo-Controlled Clinical Trial," *Lancet* 357 (2001): 251–56; K. Palvelka et al., "Glucosamine Sulfate Use and Delay of Progression of Knee Osteoarthritis: A 3-Year, Randomized, Placebo-Controlled, Double-Blind Study," *Arch Intern Med* 162 (2002): 2113–23.

12. G. Rovetta et al., "A Two-Year Study of Chondroitin Sulfate in Erosive Osteoarthritis of the Hands: Behavior of Erosions, Osteophytes, Pain and Hand Dysfunction," *Drugs Under Experimental Clinical Research* 36 (2004): 111–16.

13. Park, *Voodoo Science,* 51.